Yogini

Unfolding the
Goddess Within

Shambhavi Lorain Chopra

wisdom
tree

First published 2006
Reprinted 2007, 2008, 2009, 2010, 2011, 2012, 2013, 2014

ISBN: 978-81-8328-035-8

Published by
Wisdom Tree
4779/23, Ansari Road
Darya Ganj, New Delhi-110002
Ph.: 23247966/67/68
wisdomtreebooks@gmail.com

Printed in India

Foreword

There are many books on *Tantra* published in the world today. Most play upon either *Tantra* as sex or *Tantra* as involving strange magical practices. Few address the deeper aspects of *Tantra* or *Tantra* as a *sadhana* or spiritual path. Those that attempt this, generally just repeat the same ideas found in old *Tantric* texts, missing out on the drama, beauty and play of living *Tantra*. There is very little through which real *Tantra* can come alive and communicate to us through our own life experience. Shambhavi has provided an alternative to this — a glowing presentation of the human, naturalistic and yogic sides of *Tantra*, all woven together into her fascinating life-journey of transformation.

My contact with Shambhavi proceeded through an unusual channel. I received a letter from the great Indian scholar, Lokesh Chandra in December 2004, requesting to meet me during my next trip to Delhi. I had seen him several times before and was always eager to hear his profound remarks, not only on Indian culture but also on the state of the world. Curiously the letter arrived though it was only marked — David Frawley, Santa Fe, New Mexico, USA on the postmark! In it he mentioned a woman named Lorain Chopra, who also wanted to see me during my next trip to Delhi. He gave me her e-mail as a means of communicating with him as he had none of his own, and so our destinies crossed.

When I came to Delhi the following March, my host B.M. Thapar arranged a gathering and invited Lokesh, Lorain and a number of other friends for a visit. This was my first encounter with Shambhavi. She mentioned her interest in *Tantra*, specifically my book, *Tantric Yoga and the Wisdom Goddesses*, and gave me some of her own writings to look at. We arranged to meet privately later on so that I could give her my ideas about them.

Reading her writings, I was quite surprised. Many people approach me with writings on various subjects, particularly in India, but the writing is often poorly done or the subject is rather abstruse and of limited interest. I try to be kind to them but it is not common that one meets with someone who has a deep and natural expression, as was her case, which one can really respond positively to.

Shambhavi's writings were very fresh, direct, insightful and a joy to read. Her language was quite clear and modern and she could communicate well with a wide range of readers.

We met several times more during my stay in Delhi. Each time she brought me one or two other items. Clearly she had many of these articles. She mentioned she was writing a book, but I had no idea that it was already nearly complete.

After I returned to America, she continued to send more and more of her writings. She had not only an entire book but her very own style and cadence of expression that was unique and engaging. This was not the usual, dry, scholarly *Tantra* or the naïve personal experiences that one often reads or hears about; it was a presentation of *Tantra* that was at once profound, personal, aesthetic and adventurous. It was not an imaginary novel but her own experiences that were often more interesting than what novelists write about. Naturally I was happy to write a foreword for her, when she made this request of me some time later.

A real experience of *Tantra* is not just a *Tantric* encounter group, or getting a *Tantric* guru to chant *mantras* to help one out with one's difficulties in life. It consists of a direct contact with the *Tantric* deities and their energies as living powers, both within and around us. It requires working with the forces of Nature as powers of consciousness, discovering the *shakti* or spiritual energy in life behind all that we see and experience.

Tantric *sadhana* is a *sadhana* of life and Nature. It does not occur anywhere apart from one's daily life or apart from the natural world around us. It is a blending of our own nature with the greater cosmic Nature. It is not a purely human experience but integrates the human experience into the greater cosmic dance.

The key to *Tantra* lies in the *Tantric* deities, the forms of Shiva and Shakti as the cosmic masculine and feminine forces. Yet these *Tantric devatas* are not simply gods and goddesses made in the human form. They are our own inner divinity in its universal expression, of which our human form is but a metaphor. They are not just psychological symbols, as many thinkers like to make them out today, but existential powers and presences that dwarf the human and put our entire psychology to rest.

Shiva is the mountain and *shakti* is the mountain stream as much as they are the human male and female. Yet these forces are one. We as human beings are also the mountain and the mountain stream, the root of the tree (Shiva) and its leaves, flowers and fruit (*shakti*). Our humanity is a mask for our universality, in which exists our true being beyond birth and death.

Tantra discovers the Divine in life, in the *rasas* or essences of beauty and feeling that all our experiences are seeking. It is an alchemic process, a process of distilling the light out of darkness, which fills everything with colour. *Tantra* means the fabric of what life is woven of. It is these *rasas* that are the threads out of which our life experience is woven, and which link the outer world of our experience to the inner realms of energy and awareness from which it arises, embracing all that is and is not.

Tantra is about awakening energy at a higher level, frequency and velocity. It is about balance; not as a cancelling out of forces, but as a profound union that produces a higher life, meaning and way of expression. In this *Tantric* process, different goddesses have their important roles. Kali unfolds the transformative forces of time and space, time as the creative flow of transformation and space as the womb or matrix of new energies. She sets our *sadhana* in motion and keeps it going with her relentless force that is at times almost overwhelming.

...ara takes us from one new level of experience to another, allowing us to ascend to higher and higher planes, breaking through obstacles and boundaries, and removing negative energies with her *rudra* force. Bhairavi raises the *kundalini* or fire energy from the root *chakra* below, to rush impetuously upward with indomitable force. Sundari provides the bliss and the descending flow of *soma* from the crown *chakra*, the *ananda* that is the very *rasa* of our path, and which softens the ascending fire and allays all fears.

The goddesses are the *mahavidyas* or great forms of knowledge because they signify wisdom that arises through the cosmic energies of life, not the knowledge found in books. They are that knowledge which integrates and transforms, not which merely analyses and informs. Shambhavi relates her experiences with many of these great goddesses and shows how they can work within us. She brings them alive for us and allows us to see them with our human eyes.

Shiva is the ground of the experiencer who does not change but witnesses all changes. Shakti dances on the ground of Shiva, which is infinite space. Shambhavi weaves her experiences of Shiva into those of the *devis*, showing how both interrelate and reinforce one another.

Of the two main great traditions of India, *Tantra* and *Veda*, both are one in nature and in *mantra*. The *Veda* reflects Jyotirmaya Deva, the God of Light like the Vedic deities of fire, lightning, Sun and Moon (Agni, Indra, Surya and *Soma*). *Tantra* reflects the Shaktimaya Devi, the Goddess of Energy. But the *shaktis* are the powers of light, the electrical, magnetic, solar, lunar, lightning, dawn and fire forces. In the *Tantric* approach I work with, based upon the teachings of the great Yogi Ganapati Muni, Ramana Maharshi's chief disciple, we see *Tantra* and *Veda* as one. I find this connection in Shambhavi's work as well. She touches on the Vedic vision in her *Tantric* explorations quite naturally.

Yoga in the deeper sense is also inherently *Tantra*, an integration of the forces that weave the fabric of our lives. Similarly *Tantra* is inherently yoga or inner integration. *Tantra* provides a form and a vehicle for these powers of yoga, making them out of the dry field of mere techniques and personal strivings, into tools of worship, adoration and exaltation beyond the mind and ego.

Shambhavi, as in the Shambhavi *mudra* in which one keeps one's eyes open outwardly but directs one's attention within – it is the inner gaze of Shiva as it opens new worlds within and turns the outer world into an inner experience. It is the open 'third eye' that when seeing nothing, sees all. From that inner eye, the *shakti* arises as the lightning of perception that energises all the forces of light from the fire within the Earth to the Sun in heaven above.

Shambhavi presents us the narrative of her inner experience in a direct and flowing manner. There is no division of life and *sadhana*, inner or outer experience, her personal and her spiritual life. This allows a magic to enter into her life that we can also access. Hers is the story of a *sadhaka* who has her own inner voice, energy and unique path. She is not one seeking to mould her experience after some preconceived notion, according to a technique, or by following artificial rules. She has the energy that makes techniques work but does not depend upon them. Her human element is not excluded in an effort to sound spiritual. Her human element is included in a flow that embraces both Nature and the spirit.

This is her first book but her writings reflect a maturity of expression, a distillation of ideas, and an artistic grace that one more often sees among those who have already done a lot of writing. She is able to draw the reader into her quest, as if a part of herself, which few even mature writers are able to do.

Shakti dwells everywhere in Nature. Each temple and holy site has its own *shakti* or unique power and beauty. These places can arouse various experiences inside us and direct our *sadhana* along in a way unique to each seeker. Shambhavi has reflected her own inner experiences through some of the greatest temples and pilgrimage centres in India from Jawalamukhi and Kedarnath in the Himalayas to Kamakhya in Assam in the northeast. Her story unfolds its episodes throughout the land of India, revealing the presence of the goddess that is the soul of the country and Lord Shiva; its in-dwelling spirit.

Yogini will transform your idea of *Tantra* and allow you to experience its full flowering and effulgence woven in the tapestry of all life. It will help awaken the *yoga shakti* within you, which will take you on your own inner journey to such realms that are unknown, unpredictable, magical and sublime. No doubt we will hear further from Shambhavi in the years to come as her fascinating journey continues along with the compelling inner voice that can relate it for the benefit of all.

2005   **David Frawley**

Santa Fe, New Mexico

Prologue – Epiphany

Shambhavi gathers herein the blossoms of divinity that live in the cusp of her deep being. She expresses her self-discovery in the unprocessed ore of her simple prose that enriches the mind in universality and becomes a compelling transformation of the riptide of the spiritual realm. The classical mythopoeic context of her visualisations or *sadhana* are a flood of earthly life, a flood that our minds await. She constructs metaphysics of the bridge to step to the other shore of transcendence. As we fall into the spell of her words, like a gypsy-maiden she quietly reads the lines of our palms and assures discovery of our self, of our ethical fibre that holds together our universes, and our never-ending quest for enlightenment.

Her personal experiences in the book become the surging river of contemplation, when we resolve to cross the waters and abandon the limitations of physical existence so that now and then, here and beyond, become the purest of shadows in the harmony of body and mind, stillness and movement, you and me, and the Universe and me.

Shambhavi means serenity (*sham*) and the beauty of being (*bhava*) that humans dream about. No wonder that her book is a playground of the immortals where, "earthly cares disappear like dust", in the words of a Korean inscription in the Mureung Valley of Gods. Shambhavi is the boundary between the known and the unknown. She emerges from the dynamics of her roots and visions as a *microtheos*, a 'deity in miniature'.

Independent of the textual tradition, she reincarnates an earthy self-nature of *sadhana*. As Japanese poet Saigyo says: *Hidden deep within the root lies a flower*. She incarnates the flower of this envisioned reality of the supreme Truth that must be "read by the being".

The simple grace of Shambhavi's intense and intimately personal experiences narrated in this book are Divine symbols of life. All humans are part of an inter-dependant whole of life and symbols, of contemplation and epiphanies of the Divine. Inside a tiny seed is a banyan tree as big as the one towering above in the sky: likewise are the words of Shambhavi. She has journeyed into the substantive vision within. The divine epiphanies of the goddess, of Shiva, of the *mahavidyas* and others, have sanctified her dream space.

She returns to the mundane with new eyes that rejuvenate our experiences. Her book is a rhythm that scintillates the inner steppes of the mind, brimming with light.The physical and spiritual Universe is a single home, a *uni* or single verse. There is no *inside* without an *outside*.

The flower's sacrifice ripens in the sweetness of the fruit. Shambhavi's striving ripens as the heart work of consciousness. Lord Buddha is the *ehi-sagata-vadin* who invites us, 'come, you are welcome', to this *ehi-pasika-Dhamma*, 'to see the Dhamma for yourself', in its pure and crystalline brilliance. So does she bring the pulsating radiance and beauty of our *samskara* to us.

This book is a quantum leap in consciousness. It reminds me of a 16th century screen painting at the Freer Gallery of Art, Washington DC, entitled 'Dreaming of Immortality in a Thatched Hut'. The incredible simplicity of the thatched hut is the evocative expression of the 'eyes of life'. Likewise, this book in its spontaneity is the opening of the imaginative eye in our quest of the yonder shore.

Where travellers never went is my domain
Lokesh Chandra
Padma Vibhushan

Preface

It was never my intention to write a book or to be a writer. These were originally very personal writings of my experiences with the play of Shakti, arising as inner impulses or inspirations. The current book was written during a short spell from the fall of 2004 to spring of 2005 and emerged as a single flow from my years of a deeper search and exploration and reflects several episodes from my earlier years. The inspiration to publish these came from Prof. Lokesh Chandra with whom I had shared some of my experiences.

The book follows an inner structure, order and orientation. The sequence of episodes is random in terms of time but reflects a development of inner experiences on related topics and levels. This book is not meant as an autobiography, though my life story weaves into it in various ways. The book reflects my interaction with various friends and gurus, but it is not meant as a comment on their lives or teachings. The story is about the inner life and only touches the outer life in passing as a canvas on which it can unfold.

Life doesn't always rise to our expectations, situations unfold differently than otherwise wished, love goes all awry and trust takes a backseat in our relationships — my experiences shed light on how to handle these and became an *acceptance with an open heart.* With this I learned to be open-minded and realised the perception that brings forth the serenity in knowing that every circumstance, individual or even disappointment, is unique in its own nature. Stepping aside from umpiring a situation, one acquires the art of understanding and accepting it with a certain grace.

Tantra guided me to celebrate this fearless awareness, helping me to embrace life with a fervent passion and in freeing myself from the unconscious fears and forces of insecurity, boldly awakened my Shakti energies that in their most pure expression are a form of universal enlightenment!

I never walked this path alone, for there were beautiful people who guided me down the years and gave me that push into the throes of wonderment. And my deep-felt gratitude reaches out to each of these *light-beings* as I call them, for each has their own guiding light.

- Arjun Chopra, who nurtured me from the young child-woman into the beautiful person I am today, has blessed me with two wonderful sons — Nikhil Arjun and Ishana Arjun who despite my failings as a perfect mother, love me for what I am today.
- My mother who watched the drama unfold in silent support.
- My spiritual masters who patiently moulded me with gentle care.
- Ashokaji, who taught me to enjoy the *lila* of the Mother Goddesses.
- Prof. Lokesh Chandra, without whom there would be no book and who said, "Share your experiences with the world Shambhavi!"
- Vamadeva, for allowing Shambhavi to weave her spell.
- Shambu, who pulled me through my trying times in every way with unquestioning support.
- Joseph Dumas, who was the first person to give me a peek review of what was to unfold in my spiritual life.
- Renu Narula, my beautiful clairvoyant guide for connecting with me.
- Hari, for giving me a home away from home.
- Mahajanji who lovingly guided me through my *sadhana*.
- Come Carpentier de Gordon, for being a wonderful friend.
- Anu Narula, my lawyer who was always there for me.
- Rose, for being the gentle English rose in my life.
- My friends, who believe in me.
- Shobit, my publisher who gave me this opportunity of expression through the publishing world.
- My editor, for going through the manuscript and encouraging me to complete it in such a short time.

With deep *shraddha* to my Mevlana, for unfolding the magic of it all...

I write this book for all those passionate souls who join in the heavenly *lila* of Shiva and Shakti.

Jai Ma Guru

Contents

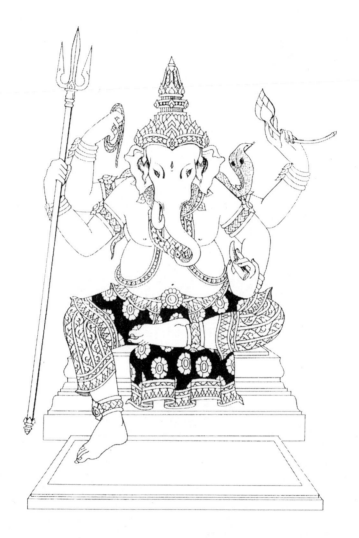

Anubhava, Inner Experience,
Leads Me to Ma Tara

The Presence of Ma Tara

'Saktivikase tu Siva eva.' - *Pratyabhijnahrdayam 13*
(On the unfolding of *shakti*, one becomes Shiva.)

At the early hour of *Brahma mahurata*, the sacred time of Brahman, on a beautiful, still dawn of the 30th day of the month of March, I woke up to the resounding, powerful vibrations of the sound *OM*... The whitewashed walls of my temple-room resonated with its reverberations. Was it a thunderous beckoning from the heavens, a shower of rain hailing springtime? The undulating *OM* sound seemed to originate from outside my window and permeated the walls, causing my entire being to quiver. I lay back, taking in this amazing current, woken abruptly from my sleep.

And there she was in her splendorous form — Goddess Tara, her *nila* (deep blue colour) skin glowing in the semi-darkness of my room. The faint light from the lit *diya* (*ghee* or clarified butter lamp) enhanced her beauty as she stood to the left side of my bed, an arm outstretched towards me, carrying a *munda*, a skull, in her palm! My body was soaked in sweat from the shock and fear of her presence. I sat up in bed and wiped the wet sweat from my neck and breasts and with a trembling hand, switched on the lamp by my bedside. The gentle strains of light from the lamp filtered through my room.

There was still a quaint trembling in my body. I found my balance and walked over to my sacred space in the corner of my room, which is my temple, and knelt before her immense presence. I lit an incense of sandalwood and prayed in silence, tears rolling down my cheeks on to my naked thighs.

I felt almost like a zombie in a trance, trying to convince myself of the beautiful *darshan* of Ma Smashan Tara — and thus began my tryst with the Dasha Mahavidya Goddesses, the Ten-Wisdom Goddesses, and my whole life began to metamorphose. The realisation of all my years of passionate *sadhana* seemed to be manifesting itself. My need to delve even deeper into experiencing *Tantra*, through meditation, *mantra yoga*, and *bhakti yoga* was beginning to make its mark on my inner process.

And life was falling in love with me all over again, waking up each day to experience the ecstasy and passion in everything around me. This encounter with the goddess was a complete shift from my dalliance with Shiva, whom I had been trying to woo through intense *bhakti* for several years.

One afternoon, while stilling myself through meditation, I sought guidance from the Divine powers to clearly show me the day when Ma would begin to connect with me. I asked my pendulum, "Show me a number when Ma will appear to me!" The answer was '9', the ninth of April 2003! My mind began calculating, realising the significance of this date. The entire configuration added up to a count of 9 (9. 4. 2003), which happened to be the date of the spring Navaratri and my destiny number. The same day a psychic, whom I met, asked me to wear a *nava-muhki* (nine-faceted) *rudraksha* bead, which is ascribed to Goddess Durga, on my left arm. The journey was on!

Navaratri Nights Invoke
Ma Durga

'Namo namo Durge sukh karni, namo namo Ambe dukh harani.'
-Durga Chalisa: 1
(I bow to You, O Goddess Durga, the bestower of all happiness.
I bow to You, O Goddess Amba, who removes all our miseries.)

Navaratri literally translates into 'nine nights'. These nine nights are devoted to the worship of Shakti wielding the power of 10 arms in the form of Durga. Each hand carries a deadly weapon of destruction bestowed on her by the gods of Hindu mythology, on the occasion of her battle against evil. Durga is known through her many forms as Kali, Bhavani, Amba and Chandika.

The *kamandal* (water-pot) that she carries in her hand was bestowed on Durga by Brahma, the *chakra* by Vishnu, the *trishul* by Shiva, the *vajra* (lightning) by Indra, the *kuthar* (axe) by Vishwakarma, the *kaladanda* (rod) by Yama, the *naga* (serpent) by Vasuki, the *kharga* and *dhal* (shield) by Surya, and the *dhanuswar* (bow and arrow) by Vayu. It is said that Durga's weapons become effective when certain *mantras* are recited by persons seeking her protection.

We all seek protection — from the mother's womb to a mother's shelter, a hand to hold while walking down a dark street, a man's reassuring hug, the warmth of a woman's bosom, Nature's gentle embrace and the Mother Goddess's protective feminine force. Life's ways never cease to create a sense of fear, even in the bravest of us. I have felt the cold chill crawl up my spine, sensing another presence in close proximity to me, as well as the fear of an impending physical assault, leaving one cowering for shelter.

These feelings of fear gradually faded away on turning to Divine grace for protection. I used *mantras* to invoke the protective powers of the magnanimous feminine force of Durgatarini and Ma Kali. My *aghora mantras* made me fearless against all the powers of darkness.

Chamunda Devi will protect us from all external harm with the ferocity of a tigress guarding her cubs. The vibrational armour of her *mantras* protects us against the shooting arrows of negative thoughts or circumstances of all kinds.

Durga accepts all the flowers offered by her devotees, but the red rose or the red hibiscus is most dear to her. There is also the tradition of offering 108 lotuses to her during the daily *puja*. In my *japa* at night, I would offer a rose petal with each *mantra* used to invoke her. Red is her colour; it is the colour of passion, love, energy, vigour, valour, and intensity of devotion.

The Navaratri is celebrated twice a year. The first is during the bright two weeks of the *Shukla Paksha* (waxing Moon) of the lunar month of *Ashwin*, occurring in September or October, the autumn. The second is during the first nine days of the bright two weeks of the *Shukla Paksha* of the lunar month of *Chaitra*, occurring in mid-March to mid-April, the springtime. For devout Shakti worshippers, these days are the most sacred. It is during these nights that Ma can most easily be invoked as it is in this period in which she grants all boons, removes negative *karmas* and bestows a prosperous and trouble-free life on her devotees.

These nine nights are dedicated to the three specific forms of the goddess — Parvati, Lakshmi and Saraswati. During the first three nights, one worships the goddess of 'action' and 'energy' through her different manifestations of Kumari, Parvati and Kali. For our spiritual self to evolve, we must first allow the attachments to our material nature to be destroyed, relinquishing all opinions, identities and beliefs. Only the sacrifice of our own ego can truly deliver us beyond every bond of ignorance and suffering. Ma Kali is the form of Divine energy and she accepts this offering willingly!

Goddess Lakshmi is worshipped for the next three nights in her various aspects of peace, abundance, bliss, fertility, love, devotion and beauty. She is the great mother in her role of fulfilling all desires and the blossoming of Divine grace and love.

The four hands of Ma Lakshmi symbolise that she has the power to bestow on us all the four aims of human life. In one hand she holds a lotus flower, reminding us of a never-ending life and the permanence of the soul. The second hand holds another lotus symbolising detachment from worldly power or *maya*. Another hand blesses everyone with wealth and abundance. The fourth hand is open and points towards the Earth, giving us support. The lotus is a symbol of unfoldment, representing the opening of the heart *chakra*.

On Lalita Panchami, the fifth day, one invokes the blessings of Saraswati, the Goddess of Knowledge. It is a time for the artist within each individual to lay down his tools before the goddess and seek her higher benediction for deeper artistic skills. She bestows spiritual knowledge that ultimately frees us from the bind of *maya*, the forces of the material world. She is worshipped during the last three days of the Navaratri. On the eighth and ninth days, *yagnas* are performed in a final act of farewell and thanksgiving.

The nine nights allow us to revel in the knowledge of the Goddess of Wisdom, invoking the deeper forces within each one of us. By imbibing their spiritual energy and power, they lead us to liberation from mire and *maya* of this worldly existence. To honour these nights is to make the entire year sacred.

My Nine Celestial Nights

'Shree Bhairava Tara jag tarini,
Chhinna bhal bhav dukh nivarini.' - Durga Chalisa, shloka 16
(It is you who redeems the world, appearing in the form of Shree
Bhairavi, Tara Devi and Chhinnamasta Devi, ending
all sorrows.)

My life became a 'nine-night wonder'. It was the first time I kept the fasts with intense passion and ardour. I went into isolation and silence, confining myself to my sacred space, praying throughout the day and during the nights and performing intense *mantra japa* and rituals. It is a period of strict fasting when only particular foods can be consumed, excluding whole grains, lentils and most of the vegetables.

It includes a beautiful ritual that is most dear to my heart — growing barley seeds in a small earthen pot filled with sand. We offer prayers to the pot, which is instilled with the life of the Mother Goddess. The growth of 'barley' is the expression of Divine Mother Earth and her grace bestowed upon us. We nurture this growth as the form of *shakti*, which takes on the vibrations of our fervent love and prayers offered to the goddess. My barley seeds grew in sheer abundance to a height of two feet, really lush and dark green.

During the Navaratri we worship the *ghata*, the earthen 'pot'. The pot is infused with *shakti* in a procedure known as *ghatasthapana*, simply meaning establishing the energy in the pot. The filling of the pot with water represents filling of the human head and making it receptive to draw *shakti* into it. The worship of this pot makes the human mind resolute, filling it with energy to bring about steadfastness in our *sadhana*.

The *jyot*, the pure oil lamp, is kept lit continuously for nine days. Ma Tara would gently bring me back to consciousness by awakening me, whenever the flickering light seemed prepared to snuff out due to the oil being got over or the wick burning out. She always amazed me by making me care for the light. On the first day of the Navaratri, I woke up to sounds of thunder and lightning early in the morning as Ma Tara appeared. I cried out, "Ma, make me strong enough to withstand your vibrations so that I can experience your beautiful self!" The lamp suddenly went out and darkness enfolded me. I lay back, closing my eyes in a mesmerised state, when suddenly she held my right foot and lifted it nearly two feet into the air. Waking up from my state of reverie, I relit the lamp.

I began to carry the earthen bowl of barley seeds outside, prepared very lovingly for germination. The moment I stepped on to the terrace, I raised my glance to the night sky. Just overhead, a solitary small dark cloud appeared and large raindrops begin to fall on my face. Lifting my arms high above me, raising the barley to the sky, my heart cried out, for undeniably I was left spellbound! I received Ma's blessings in the form of raindrops that would gently fall down on me and then suddenly stop, with the cloud vanishing equally suddenly. I would come inside and quietly sit and pray. This phenomenon continued every dawn of the Navaratri. I talked to my other friends about this but they said that they saw no clouds or rain on these mornings.

On the fourth day of the Navaratri, at night, I awoke to the footfalls of an animal — the distinct clicking of uncut, overgrown nails of a dog to the right side of my bed. A black dog of no particular breed, short and longish in stature, was walking past. The door to my room was shut and there seemed no way anything could have entered. I could sense there was a definite cosmic Divine play going on between Shiva and His consort. At dawn, the same morning, I heard a soft whisper in the most melodious feminine voice, "Wake up!" This was followed by

bot of an owl right outside my window. I wasn't aware of ever
 ̣g heard an owl in the vicinity before. In his fierce form as *Bhairava*,
Shiva's mount (*vahana*) is the black dog, befitting the archetypal image
of this shamanic God.

On the fifth day, there was a knock on the door at the dark hour
before dawn. Rushing to open the door in a sleepy stupor, I realised it
was only Ma awakening me for her next day. Throughout the fifth,
sixth and seventh days, I awoke to the continuous hooting of the owl.

Sitting before my altar, I saw Ma Durga astride a tiger superimposed
on Shiva with a luminous white light emanating all around him, holding
me spellbound. In *Tantra*, such superimposition is referred to as *bindu
bheda*, when the pupils of both eyes become centred together, and two
separate figures are made to merge into one. The *bindu bheda* is a
necessary preliminary step to the practice of *shambhavi mudra*, a state
that can bring about a spontaneous meditative union with the Supreme
Shiva.

I was fighting for my sanity, questioning the reality of what was
happening around me. All this wasn't occurring in my dreams. It was
unfolding during my waking moments. One night over the phone, I
asked, "Am I going crazy, Gurudeva?" He reassured me that I was
not. He said that these inner experiences would even come more often
and I should not be afraid of them, using the help of my *guru mantra*.

He explained various practices to intensify my *sadhana*, following
certain simple rituals. He beautifully expressed how Shiva was always
static and could only be experienced through his *shakti*. The 'white light'
that I was seeing, he said, represents a *sattvic*, pure nature. Overcome
with deep emotion, tears flowed down my cheeks; so much seemed to
be happening which was far beyond my reasoning capacity at times.

At the same hour of dawn on day eight, I awoke to the gentlest
sprinkle of water on my face, for Ma is ever so playful with her children.
Sitting in meditation to the hooting of the owl, her presence became
very powerful. I began to desire her *darshan* more than ever. My need
for her beautiful face to appear became an obsessive passion. Sages
say that she offers her devotee the entire cosmos to make sure that no

desires are left unfulfilled. The eighth day is very auspicious: Durga Ashtami, the day of appearance of the incarnation of Shakti in the human form. It is the night when we must get connected to her, for she will clear us of our *karmic* debts.

I isolated myself from the world in silent spells of no communication, consciously striving to raise my vibrational levels. To connect with the higher powers during *sadhana*, we need to extricate ourselves from external time and space and enter instead the mythic time and space of the goddesses.

During this Navaratri I lost nine kilos of weight and my mother became anxious about the change. Initially she was wary of my *sadhana*, unable to relate to the deities herself. She would cause ripples, be it concerning my involvement in prayers or the dogs in the home not being allowed to have their non-vegetarian meals. Yet, it was really only during the Navaratri, which came twice a year, that I followed such restrictions.

In the beginning, I guess my *sadhana* wasn't strong enough as I would get easily disturbed at my mother's comments. A *sadhak*-friend explained to me that by such reactions, all my nine days of *sadhana* could become futile. Gradually I prayed for her also to keep the peace. Wonderfully, a time soon came when she would light the incense and lamp before my deities; even bathe and dress them for me.

Ma Tara kept appearing to me every day, her actions differing each time. It was her way of drawing me into her fold. I was beginning to accept Ma in her various forms. She no more seemed to terrify me with her powerful presence, unlike the first time when she drove me into a profuse sweat of intense fear.

During the eighth night, she appeared with the *khand*, a weapon in the shape of a head chopper, and in one sweep, she swiftly drove it through the centre of my head but without spilling a drop of blood. Later, I was explained, this was her way of making me deal with my 'ego-self'. To be without a head is a yogic metaphor for reaching beyond body consciousness or attachment to the thought compositions of the mind.

11

Each experience occurred with a perfect clarity of vision, action, colour and minute details that my memory recorded with great precision. There was a sharp difference between experiencing and dreaming. The dreams seemed unclear and faded quickly away from my conscious mind, while my experiences remained etched in stone. I'd ink them down with calligraphic flourishes in my little notebook. To invoke Ma, I would fervently and tirelessly worship her. I knew she would never forsake her loving *sadhakas*.

My path is one of an *anubhavi*, an inner experiencer. I wanted to explore and directly experience what I had read and learnt. This adds a dimension of practical value or else the knowledge gained remains borrowed. Whether it comes from the scriptures or from people's lives, it is always limited to another's experience or presentation. My entire faith was built around what had unfolded within me. I couldn't propound any faith or doctrine that I hadn't actually experienced. I was determined to figure out the real energies existing in the cosmos.

I followed my path in a systematic manner, listening to my inner voice. This began after extricating myself from a marriage of 15 years. The next process began with an intense purification of the body, mind and soul through *mantra japa*, which paved the way for a deeper understanding of *bhakti*.

I wanted to place myself completely at Shiva's feet and my path to be directed through His grace. I found it much easier to surrender to one's personal deity in a visualised form than to surrender to some abstract cosmic energy. The vastness of the cosmos perplexed me at times. I wanted to pour my passionate love into one point, instead of dissipating it in different directions. It is much easier to love and worship a deity like Ma or Shiva.

Of all the various forms of worship, I believed the surest way was mental worship, having had no traditional Vedic background and realising that physical or ritualistic worship is always limited. To avoid the possibility of a mistake in performing a ritual or pronunciation of a *mantra*, I tried to internalise my energies through mental worship.

Experiencing pain, anger, and distrust in all its intensity is never easy. It is always difficult; the easier path being to live a life of convenience and pulling blinkers over one's eyes. Most of the times we go on avoiding our own deep-set miseries. In a bid to escape the present, we lose ourselves to the temptations of shopping, watching television, running in and out of social events and relationships. We try to keep away from the true 'inner self' and camouflage our hurt inside. Most people go on avoiding their inner selves.

My mind was made up — I'd go into the suffering, feel the hurt, feel the pain, and experience the anguish. Unless we go deep into our suffering, we cannot be released from life's imprisonment. By fully experiencing an emotion, we learn to absorb it. We become aware that emotions are located not only in the heart, but in every part the body. Negative emotions affect the entire body and eventually manifest in some form of ailment.

I made myself stronger in order to experience the suffering — accepting it, welcoming it and feeling grateful for it. I learned that when one's own suffering is fully experienced and absorbed willingly, it comes to manifest as a blessing. The same energy stored as hatred can be turned into love; pain within us becomes a pleasure and suffering transforms into bliss.

Yet nothing seemed to flow easily for me — moving through a gamut of shortcomings, minor tribulations, misunderstandings, and insecurities, I was truly put to the grindstone by the higher forces. I held on to a deep faith in mankind, despite all else, evolving through my daily life situations. Trust played a significant role. I placed more trust into my relationships, gave more opportunities for the other person to reveal who they are, sometimes even giving them enough rope to hang themselves! At least I tried to learn my lessons and prayed dearly to be released from ordinary *karmic bandhans*, so I could move on with my journey.

Slowly the healing process began and since then I never looked back at either the relationships or at the situations. The poison that I had swallowed eventually proved to become the nectar for a higher life! I was happier in every manner! Ma showed me all this by the end of the nine nights.

Healing the Anguish

'Prem bhakti se jo yash gavey, dukh-daaridra nikat nahin aavey.'
- Durga Chalisa v. 27
(The one who sings your glory with devotion, love and sincerity is
beyond the reach of grief and difficulties.)

The cosmic consciousness of the Universe can heal us. There is a
deep cry arising from each soul for global healing, for a healing
light to pervade our darkness. We all need to heal as a consequence of
the ravages of society and our own mindset. We have been deeply
disturbed and our vibrations have been reduced to negativity of gross
macro levels. Love is the highest and purest form of healing. Healing
is a spontaneous outpour of loving energy brought about by one's
desires and intentions.

I had just violently removed myself from a painful emotional
situation that in today's world is not uncommon — a man breaking
your deep trust and dallying with your close companion. I still find it
hard to call her my friend, though I have healed from the situation,
running away from it initially and learning to deal with it finally.

One very early morning, though to me it was still the dark night,
Kunti aggressively shook me and said, "Wake up, I have something to
tell you." She was still reeling from the three-fourths of a bottle of rum
that she had consumed. She looked menacingly at me; my calm
composure always seemed to ruffle her disturbed soul. With the

choicest of *gaalis* (abuses), the lucid abusive language of north India, she poured out her gory little story. I was in shock, not only at her dalliance, but with her it seemed to be how she conducted her life as I had witnessed earlier. I had moved away from being judgmental of people. I came to understand that each person has his or her own reasons for the action he or she performs. The humiliation of the entire relationship had left me deeply scarred. Nevertheless, deep anguish can lead one to a path of profound inner search.

Taking a flight to Hyderabad, a new phase began in my life. Mithoo had remained a dear friend through my college days. Amidst the celebrations of her daughter's wedding, a most beautiful actress named Amla came my way. I guess she had been through her own trials and tribulations and was now using the meditative form of Vipassana to heal her soul. She also knew the art of regression, where through meditation and gentle hypnosis we can go back into an earlier lifetime.

Somehow Amla agreed to do a past-life regression with me, but only after she extracted a promise that I would go in for the 10-day Vipassana course. The promise was given and she took me back into another world; a world where I contacted my maternal grandmother, a beautiful, very gentle soul who left her body at a young age.

Closing my eyes in gentle meditation, my consciousness was suddenly transferred to the body of a beautiful woman dressed in flowing white robes, caught up at the breasts and high waist, with flowing dark hair and barefoot. Nana, as we lovingly addressed my grandmother, was comforting me, and leading me through tall woods where I lived in a quaint wooden cottage. Surrounded by Nature's abundance, in the solace of quietude, a deep tranquillity prevailed around me.

I regressed further to the day of my leaving the body in that life. We reached a point where running softly, barefoot through the woods, in the distance I could hear Amla's gentle voice asking me if I was fleeing in fear. Somehow I never felt any fear. There was a freedom of abandonment to the vastness of Nature. What was I running from? Where was I running?

Gentle tears began to roll down my cheeks and a constriction appeared in my throat. Pain has a prodding way of bringing to consciousness one's anguish. At last, had the footsteps of mysterious death caught up with me? I began a struggle with my consciousness, when Amla decided to bring me back to the waking state. Maybe I wasn't ready to witness the end in an earlier life.

After the session, a sense of lightness came into my being, as if I had dealt with all the pain and anguish. My days through the wedding festivities drew to a close and I flew back to Delhi. I went in for my 10-day Vipassana retreat, having been warned that it would not be easy on my being, but that I was to stay on as per my promise made.

Vipassana is a technique of truth-realisation, self-realisation, delving into the reality of what one calls 'oneself', and in a way becomes a tool for God-realisation. After all, God is nothing but truth, love and purity. Every time an impurity arises in the mind, such as fear, anger, and hatred, one becomes miserable and agitated. Whenever something untoward happens, we become tense and begin tying knots in our mind and body. Throughout life one repeats this process until the entire mental and physical being is a bundle of Gordian knots. To learn the art of living harmoniously, one must first find the cause of disharmony, and the cause always lies within us. We need to explore the true reality of this deep inner self.

The simplicity of the programme humbled me and the rigidity in the time schedule taught me discipline. Vipassana involved a strict code of discipline, which included *ahimsa*, vegetarianism, and avoidance of intoxicants, celibacy and total silence. The long hours of meditation on the breath and scouring the sensations in every part of the body honed my faculty of observation. Through understanding the phenomenon of impermanence within the body, I learnt to centre the mind in equanimity. By the fifth day of meditation, both my body and will power were beginning to give way. I was caving in; all the gross emotions were racking my being, the past bringing in its wake intense pain and anguish in its wake of memories.

'Would I have the courage to pull through? O Lord, give me the necessary strength to bear the onslaught of this intense negativity, manifesting itself in pain. Help me keep up my promise to Amla.' On day six of the Vippassana course, my reserves of strength had dwindled to an all-time low, and my nerves were frayed. The *maun vrat*, the vow of absolute silence, the isolation, the meditational process of 'looking within the self', missing my sons, my heartache — all seemed to take their toll on me.

By evening, an excruciating pain was experienced, incomparable to even the labour pains experienced during the birth of both my sons. It was as if a sword heated through burning embers was driven through my back and the heart *chakra*. The severity of the pain rendered me unable to even sit up. In sheer weakness of will, I approached the *sadhaka* in charge, a gentle German girl, and explained my situation to her with minimal words, "I can't take this any more; the pain is so excruciating that it won't let me sit through the evening. May I please rest my back against the wall?"

"Shambhavi, this technique is working for you. Trust me, this too shall pass. You must go through with it; we cannot allow you to change your position or rest against the wall."

I will never know how I managed to sit through the last phase of the evening, with the pain singeing my being. Retiring to the confines of my room that night, I threw myself on to the bed and wept shamelessly, my body writhing in the raging fire, till I was exhausted and lulled by the pain I fell into the arms of Morpheus. Suffering and pain seemed to act like 'sandpaper', redefining my inner being.

Paradoxically, sometimes I viewed it as a great gift, but this was only much later. Suffering is with God's (Shiva's) consent. Our acceptance of suffering is our gift to Him. It is also through faith in His power and His grace that we are able to accept the suffering He allows. He knows why He gives suffering and when He will take it away. It is through trust in His love that we bear the suffering in peace and with dignity.

Waking up the next morning, feeling as light as a feather, the first soft hues of the Sun's rays played on my face through the window. I stepped out of bed, feeling like a child. I was late for my early morning meditation, but the German girl caught my eye and smiled gently. She knew I had survived the trauma of my *karmas* and had emerged a winner. This is what life is all about — being a winner at the core. To me life is always beautiful. The trials and tribulations, pain and anguish are part of the *karmic* cycle. It is how we accept the reality, acknowledge it and gracefully move on that make us a winner.

Vipassana taught me the art of humility and the importance of the word 'equanimity' — the quality of being calm and even-tempered. Down the line, it made it easier for me to learn to forgive and thereby to let-go! Most importantly, if one wants to progress spiritually, the art of forgiveness has to be learned on the deepest levels and only then we can let go.

Those of us who dare to venture on a different path will pay the price for being different, for thinking differently and living life on an experiential level. Spirituality is a love affair — a love affair with existence. The waves of spirituality arise in awe and wonder, and in feeling this we experience divinity but not just by reading the scriptures and listening to holistic discourses.

The Play of Light

'Noor – e – Ellahi'
(The brilliant play of light.)

On the seventh morning of the Vipassana session, having been calmed after my intensely painful experience, I began to feel forceful vibrations, like a flow of energy playing around me. Opening my eyes in the dimly lit hall, through a tiny opening in the centre of the dome-shaped roof, a flow of light, scintillating and quivering pencilled rays of sunshine poured down on me. My being felt a loss of physical weight, a floating sensation.

Taking in the luminosity of space, oblivious to everything around me, I was wonderstruck, and in an instant the rays vanished. And resuming my meditation with a serene stillness, I fell in sync with everyone. The experience was gently described to me by an elderly person meditating in the room. He came up to me after the programme, when we were allowed to speak. He described the entire picturesque effect of the play of light on me that he had seen.

Both the realms of light and of darkness are of a higher dimension, meeting at a single point, which is the Earth. This is the reason we experience both the Divine and the demonic forces on the Earth. Forces from both hemispheres are incarnating as human beings.

The term 'higher dimensions' refers to parallel worlds, from the lower Earth-bound astral worlds of 'dark' forces to the much higher worlds of light beings. These forms or forces are not perceivable to the physical eye, as they vibrate at different wavelengths. Matter is nothing but vibrations of energy, including higher 'invisible' cosmic energies, known to only to a few earthly beings. Many of these invisible beings, though not all, are angelic with an aura of Divine harmony.

People with a completely materialistic bent of mind can only conceive what they see with their eyes. The human mind is capable of destroying its environment to fulfil its selfish needs, creating a cruel war industry, delving in unethical politics, and projecting a future world based on sheer destruction. Definitely, people who do this belong to the dark forces, which initially listen to the commands of the 'man' trying to control them, but at some point of time the same man becomes his own victim, coming under their control instead.

The human being who works with the spirit to fulfil the aims of the ego is practicing a form of black magic. He may temporarily gain something from this 'connection', but eventually he will face destruction from the same force. The forces working through these dimensions or 'other worlds' can either be God-conscious beings of light, which some refer to as angels, or the beings of darkness referred to as 'fallen angels'. Others may call them *devas* and *asuras*. But the really higher powers cannot be reached through such manipulations.

We must realise certain basic truths in order to avoid these dark pitfalls. God is Absolute. In reality, there are no devils or evil forces that could ever contend with the Absolute. God is clearly beyond all negative and positive aspects, such as we see in the symbolism of Shiva. Some so-called servers of God have created a manic state of fear in our minds using words like 'Satan' or the 'devil' to intimidate their subjects, generally into doing what they want.

Clairvoyant people, who are able to perceive subtle material energies, acknowledge that negative forces can affect only those individuals who are open to such resonances. No evil force can bother any human being who does not vibrate with the same frequency. The person against whom evil forces are projected in black magic will be affected only to the extent that he too vibrates on the same levels. If one is not open to such forces, the evil vibrations will bounce back to the person sending them and with an even more powerful force.

The Absolute is beyond any form of duality as he is omnipresent and omnipotent, the Divine reality. Our goal towards the creation of a harmonious world is to become Divine ourselves and to perceive a higher consciousness in all relative situations, understanding both the good and the bad experiences, realising our true spiritual nature beyond them.

Spiritual Healing

'Aum hrim shrim klim adya kalika param Eshwari svaha.'
(*Aum* and salutations to she who is the first one, dark within her own reality, the supreme primordial feminine, who cuts through illusion to the absolute truth of existence.)

Through my mystical experiences, certain changes began to occur in my life and new potentials to arise, taking me to higher levels of action and expression. Inner energies would manifest to heal the body, mind and soul, paving the way for a happy and higher living. There were no rules necessary for raising one's vibrations to subtler levels, sharpening one's intuition, honing one's finer skills, listening to the inner voice and living in harmony with cosmic vibrations. It happened through its own inner impulse.

In spiritual healing, we play with subtle energies. Most eastern medicinal systems have acknowledged and used such forces since Vedic times, and now Western medicine is recognising their importance as well. The unity of the self and the world is the ultimate aim of our existence. Self–realisation helps us refine the soul, liberating and humanising the systems we work with in our surroundings — be it in our personal life, politics or business.

I explored various methods to heal my inner self. These included prayer, channelling of spiritual energy or *prana*, *Chi*, Reiki, healing or protecting oneself through visualisations, advanced levels of concentration, developing psychic abilities and cultivating universal compassion.

My deepest experience was to acknowledge the problem and the deep pain, understanding and being one with it, not necessarily having to approve of it. One must experience life fully, realising that pain and pleasure are intrinsic aspects of our lives, coexisting with the forces of Nature. We need to empathise with the person who has hurt us, understanding the intensity of his or her own individual predicament. Praying for his or her spiritual sustenance, making a wish to take on his or her suffering, visualising some of the other person's anguish — these are all different ways to help relieve the other of a portion of his or her individual pain.

This was never easy for me. I had to muster up a lot of empathy. Taking on some of his or her suffering, one also gives him or her some of one's own happiness to help the person through his or her strife. One can visualise his or her problems or pain being taken into our heart *chakra* as a black smoke and simultaneously goodwill and happiness from our heart will flow out to the person in the form of white light. The black smoke can be used to help us destroy our own pain, confusion and problems as well, replacing it with our own white light. This should in the final analysis lead to a feeling of joy and peacefulness.

A Psychic Experience
with Death

'You would know the secret of death.
But how shall you find it unless you seek it in the heart of life?'
- Kahlil Gibran

Reiki or *pranic* healing is the energy of directly applying *Chi* for the purpose of strengthening one's aura or energy system. The energy regulates its own flow to and within the person receiving the healing, drawing through the healer exactly what is required to heal. Through Reiki everything can be healed because the only limits of Reiki are the recipient's willingness to accept the healing and change. Reiki works with the vibrations of the healing touch of Nature, the subtle cosmic energies prevailing in the Universe.

During a group discussion on past-life regression, my Reiki master, whom I had not yet met, focused his eyes on me. He was a tall, graceful Sikh, who had spent his best years sailing the high seas. Through the entire session I grew conscious of his gaze following me. We all went through our experiences of a past life, mine being a deep experience into the serpent powers of the time of the Pharaohs. Entering monumental golden gates to the kingdom of a life lived eons ago left me quite disturbed, nonetheless.

The session having ended, seemingly in a state of deep silence, the Sardar gentleman walked up to me and said, "Do you heal?" Those days I was experiencing long spells of very intense *sadhana*, literally performing my *japa*, the *mantra* recitation, throughout the day, moving into the count of lakhs. My being was going through wonderful moods, creating upheavals in my daily life.

"I see a very beautiful white aura surrounding you," he said. He was convinced that I would learn the art of healing and should begin with Reiki, inviting me to take initiation from him. He became persistent over time, calling me regularly, gently explaining the ways of Reiki.

I decided to accept the healing gift of the Universe, making Reiki a way of life. Within three days of my first-level initiation, he asked me to send some healing energy for his maid, who was unable to conceive and was having severe pains in the abdominal region. In spite of my nervousness, he gently guided me to begin. I lost myself somewhere. Suddenly powerful white rays swooping over sapphire blue, crystal waters, began to emanate from Shiva's raised hand sitting high above a mountain. The rays burned the centres of my palms. The glimmer of the light was scintillating.

My Reiki master's hand on my shoulder guided me into the presence of the moment. The master held a hand-mirror up to my face, making me see my own reflection. The effect of my face shining like the moon made me blush! The maid was in a deep slumber, her face flushed like a child bride. He wanted me to share my experience with him and said, "What were you seeing Shambhavi?" Hesitating to tell him initially, after much persuasion I did, nervous that he might ridicule me. The maid proved to have received Shiva's blessings and soon had a baby.

I became a formidable student, at times loving and deeply reverential, but also free thinking and questioning what wasn't clear to me; at times, even making strong statements. My relationship with the teacher was always woven around a certain comfort zone, creating space for individual expression, truthfulness, caring and a great sense of humour. Humour formed a wonderful basis for bonding through trust. The humour never allowed me to take myself seriously.

Breezing into his home, I would ask for coffee — one of my preferences that I never gave up, even during intense *sadhanas*. Being

A Psychic Experience with Death

Divine was not at all about depriving the self or creating suffering; it was about being ecstatically in love with every moment of life, picking up the threads of joy even after episodes of pain and anguish. That is how I survived, maintaining an inner and an outer radiance.

Working closely I sensed a lot of deep-seated anger and pain in him. One relaxed afternoon, mentioning my observation to him, he began to pour out all his setbacks. Our relationship took an interesting turn for I began to gently guide him to heal from his inner turmoil. He would lightheartedly admonish me, when I'd bully him around for a cup of coffee saying, "Who is the master here?"

Once, while away in south India, I began to receive frantic calls from my Reiki master, "Where are you? Why aren't you calling? Return immediately! I need you!" I sensed a desperate urgency in his voice and wasn't able to understand the reason why. On my last afternoon, I was extremely uneasy and upset, deeply sensing that something was going to happen to him. That evening I boarded the flight for Delhi, and remained restless throughout the night with a heaviness and slight premonition!

Early the next morning, along with the *dhotis* that my master had asked me to get for him from the south, I headed for his home. En route calling up his home, the maid answered the phone in tears, questioning me where I was. "*Saab* is not here any more. He kept asking for you." Between her sobs, I tried to get an answer on his whereabouts so early in the morning.

Death always sends you reeling! Impossible! He had suffered a heart attack and just left the clock ticking on the mantle shelf. Uncontrollable tears streamed down my face, my heart bearing the deep anguish of losing a master and a friend. Memories came rushing to my mind of the time when in exasperation he threw up his arms and took me to meet his guru. "Guruji, what do I do with this girl? I just can't handle her; so many difficult questions she throws at me." Other times he would throw back his handsomely turbaned head in a hearty laughter, his silvery mane catching tinges of light from the chandelier.

The pain of the loss brought home to me the disturbance of doubting my own sensitivity levels and the ensuing questioning of higher truths.

Why was I not able to read the urgency in his calls or sense his fear of impending death? Why could I not comfort him in his time of need? The answers to my questions were consigned to the flames that lit up his pyre.

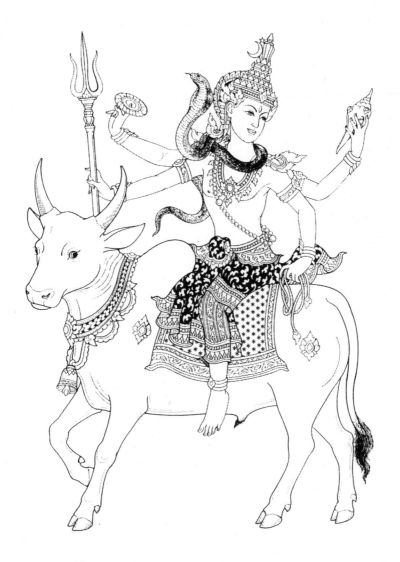

Shiva Brings Transcendence
into My Life

Shiva is Pure Existence

'Siva is pure existence, the immortal Divine principle. Siva is pure
consciousness, unconditional and transcendental; Shiva is the deity of the
manas (mind), the Lord of Yoga, master of the three worlds and the
conqueror of death. The whole Universe is created by the *shakti* of Siva.'
- *Shiva Purana*

My spiritual journey began with Dr D.V. Krishna, who translated
my *janampatri*, astrological chart, which says I was born with the
blessings of Shiva, and no matter where my life would lead me, Shiva
would search me out in this vast Universe and bring me to His feet.
His guidance set me on my path of deeply searching for Shiva. Gurudev
unravelled the mysteries that were soon to become my experiences.
He sent me completely aware on my first journey to Dharamsthala
near Bangalore, to seek Shiva's *anugraha*.

We set upon the long drive from Bangalore on an early May morning. The drive proceeded through lush, tall, green ferns reaching amazing heights of over seven feet, allowing the rays of the Sun to play with
their shadows like a meditation in itself. It had been raining heavily
and the road at one point was impossible, except for trucks, to traverse.
The driver grew apprehensive on seeing several vehicles being way-
laid. Ahead of us a truck was literally skidding off the narrow path
that was now all that remained of the road.

Praying fervently, going over my *guru-mantra*, I was seeking a way out. I was not going to turn back without paying obeisance to Lord Shiva. Obstacles will always be there. This is what my personal experiences have time and again proved. How one transcends them into workable situations is where we score the brownie points down the path of life.

Reassuring the driver that we would get through this extremely rough patch, he shot me a look that clearly said, 'you are crazy'. Putting the car into gear and giving it his all, we did get across, to everyone's surprise. I have immense faith in the ways of the Divine, despite all the difficulties having been experienced in the most trying times. We arrived at the temple and saw this long queue of endless devotees. Looking around, thinking to myself that this will take ages, a priest suddenly came up and offered to guide me into the temple sanctuary for a *darshan*.

I stood quite mute in front of the *Shivalingam* and felt strong vibrations travelling through the ground and entering my being, leaving my legs with a faint trembling. Becoming conscious of people gathering around, I went on to circumambulate the sanctum sanctorum. This is called *pradakshina*. The Lord is the centre, the very source of our existence and we must move around this focal point for His grace to flow into us.

After completion of worship, we usually circumambulate around ourselves in a clockwise direction, recognising the supreme divinity within us. Focusing on the inner divinity, the pure consciousness of the soul begins a transformation at the deepest core of the heart, leading us to awaken our spiritual purpose by creating an awareness of the prevailing cosmos.

Yogeshwar, the Celestial Yogi

'Asanasthah sukham hrade nimajjati.'
-Shiva Sutra 3.16
(The yogi who establishes himself in a steady posture
easily becomes immersed in the ocean of the heart.)

Yogeshwar is Shiva as the Lord of Yoga, the celestial ascetic, who after exploring the entire evolution of life and consciousness through the power of yoga was able to transcend all forms into the Absolute. There were certain experiences that allowed Him to do this, as reflected in various stories about Him.

Shiva retreated to Kashi. His heart was angry, sorrowful and remorseful. His hands were smeared with the blood of Brahma, the Creator, whose head He had cut off, realising that He could not find the higher truth within this manifest realm. He brooded over the questions that plagued His heart and soul and meditated on the ways to understand these disturbances and realise the truth beyond the veils of *maya*, illusion. Finally He found the way through the practice of 'yoga' — the means to yoke the individual's mind with the Supreme, where humanity and Nature can be one with the higher consciousness of the cosmos.

Under a great banyan tree, seated on a tiger skin, facing *dakshina*, the south, He revealed the knowledge of yoga without any *dakshina*, or fee, to His devotees. For this, His students called him *Dakshinamurti*, the great cosmic teacher. He explained the two realities of existence —

both eternal. One is the *purusha*, the serene cosmic spirit that stands still beyond the reach of time and space, and the other is *prakriti*, Nature, matter, the cosmic substance, the source of time and space, which is always in a state of complexity.

What is born and reborn, bringing about experiences of anguish and passion, is not the *purusha*, but the body and the mind, one's *prakriti*. We are reborn because we are attached to the world by our *samskaras* and our *karma*, and these actions generate further reactions creating further experiences, if not in this lifetime, then in another.

Yoga helps one to view the world as it really exists, with clarity, dispassion, and wisdom, through conscious awareness and not merely through opinions, emotions and preconceptions. Through yoga we can extricate ourselves from all delusions, ignorance, and attachments that bind us within the relative world, stilling the mind and remaining aware and unaffected by the existing turbulence around us. Shiva manifested His body into various *asanas*, yoga postures, depicting the movements of various birds and beasts, energising the body, revealing the pulsating animal instincts deep within man, bringing them within one's consciousness and will power.

Shiva revealed the secret of *pranayama*, breath-manipulation, of being able to control the movement of *prana*, the life-giving energy, thus enabling the mind to expand beyond the narrow confines of the body. The great sage Patanjali documented all of Shiva's profound teachings. "Go into yourself, as a turtle goes into its shell." This *pratyahara*, the internalisation or withdrawal of the mind from the sense objects, will connect the soul with experiencing the finer nuances of Nature and discovering the true cosmic reality behind all appearances.

With *dharana* (concentration) and *dhyana* (meditation), one can finally reach a state of *samadhi*, the ability to be truly objective, rising above all subjectivity — both mental and physical — and becoming one with *purusha*, the cosmic soul. Comprehending this pure existence leads to *moksha* (enlightenment), taking our awareness beyond all limitations, bringing in its wake an inner transformation, a power, a passion, a will to live the most complete and compassionate life that is possible for us.

Yoga is this process of unfolding the spiritual self, emphasising the concepts of harmony, union and the consolidation of personal traits for a higher goal. In this unfolding, breath awareness is probably the most essential tool. Breathing forms the link between the body and the mind. Breath awareness is an integral part of our being alive as well as a means of creating a higher consciousness.

Yoga is being in touch with the very pulse of the universal energies, and vibrating in tandem with their gentle throb.

'Om dakshinamurtaye namaha!'

Tattvas, the Elements, and Nature's Healing

'Om shri dhanvantaraye namaha.'
(Salutations to the celestial healer.)

The entire world is made up of the five great *tattvas* or elements of Earth, water, fire, air and ether. A sixth factor is *mahatattva* or cosmic intelligence, which, though less talked about, changes the inner dynamics of these elements through God consciousness, bringing about healing at an inner core. Everything in the manifest Universe, including we human beings, is a configuration of these five elements.

The process of *Tantra* requires the purification of the five elements in order to help the *kundalini shakti* ascend. The *kundalini* can rise only when the elements in our body are purified of their heavier accretions. All *sadhana*, meditation and yoga, involve different processes to purify these elements, aiding their flow and transformation.

Since the human body consists of a certain combination of these elements, they can be balanced in Ayurvedic medicine in order to restore our health. *Akash*, ether or space, is the subtlest of the elements. It resembles the quantum mechanical concept of the field from which all matter is created and into which all matter resolves. *Akash* is the source of all the other elements, and interacts with them through its vibrations. Sound is the quality of ether, representing an entire spectrum of vibration: audible sound, cosmic radiation, X-rays, gamma rays, ultra-violet and visible light. Ether gives us the space in which to manifest and develop.

Fasting creates an inner space, a vacancy for the body to recuperate and repair, rest and heal itself. Ayurveda has classified certain *vaigs*, movements or Nature calls, including sleep, sneeze, cough, tears and perspiration to help us work with this space, emphasising but never interfering with our natural impulses.

Space has various forms of manifestation, not just in the physical Universe, but also the space of the mind moving to higher levels, and the supreme space of pure consciousness beyond every relative manifestation.

All space has its own energy. Space is the matrix of *shakti*. Goddess Bhuvaneshvari, the infinite mother in her manifestation as the cosmic womb, is also the element of space, dwelling in the microcosmic space within the heart.

Space creates healing. By accepting the failures of my emotional experiences and the emptiness they created, I came to understand the true power of love. Love creates a supporting space, giving the loved one a freedom going far beyond the shackles of selfish desire. This beautiful space is one that nurtures and manifests as Divine love.

Agni or the fire element in *Tantra* is the origin and end of all phenomena. The sacred fire has influenced spiritual rituals and traditions since the most ancient times. Fire is both worldly and transcendental. The *Tantric* texts explain the existence of both 'inner' fire and 'outer' fire. The inner fire is the vital principle focused at the navel centre, which when stimulated by deep breathing blazes upward in the body, consuming the impurities of both mind and body. In Ayurveda, the fire in the navel is called *jatharagni*, the gastric fire that helps digest food and allows for the assimilation of life-sustaining nutrients.

Fire gives one clarity and sharpness of perception. One of the simplest ways to enhance the fire element in the body is to sunbathe for 15 to 30 minutes a day; but only in the rays of the early morning rising Sun or late afternoon setting Sun, when the sunrays fall on the body at an angle, and never vertically.

Tattvas, the Elements, and Nature's Healing

A half-hour brisk daily walk has a salutary effect on the body. After a meal, one should also take a leisurely stroll. Never bathe after a meal; it literally is like pouring water over a fire.

As an early morning ritual, after offering water to the Sun-god, I would gently drink three glasses of water, concentrating on the flow moving through my being.

Jal tattva, the water element, nourishes and sustains the spirit as well as the physical body. We must allow its flow into the psyche. The flow of water carries with it the *shakti* energies and power of life. Ganga is pure *shakti*; her energies can heal one's being and psyche. *Shakti* cannot only be found in the freedom of space but also in the free flow of water. Water nourishes the *rasa* in our being, rejuvenating our inner essence as well as creating an outer glow.

Rain-water is purifying and therapeutic in its effect. Bathing in rain-water washes away the body's negativities, bringing about a sensual flow through one's being. In our society, we must encourage natural systems of rain-water harvesting, more so in rural areas, to gain all of its benefits.

The worship of the air element can be done through the control of *prana*, the life force, as in the practice of *pranayama*. One should do this with a certain amount of caution. Many instructors today misguide the layman. One needs to be physically and mentally fit to safely practice *pranayama* in today's world. Our nervous system should not be over-stressed by the practice.

Because we live in a heavily polluted environment (where the water and air tend to be unclean) and noise, radiation, and stress surround us, our nervous system is weakened considerably. *Pranayama* done wrongly or too forcefully can disturb us further. *Pranayama* must be deeply understood by the teacher and by the student, considering the right environmental influences for it to really work.

Without *anubhava*, personal experience, one will sink into a quagmire of preachings and teachings. Accept guidance as *prasada* from the Lord, through the teacher as His instrument and experience the practice for yourself with a clear understanding. Realise that I am responsible for my own growth and must experience every reality for myself in order to reach the Divine consciousness.

Jimutavahana, Shiva Rides the Clouds

'Svecchaya svabhittau visvam unmilayati.'
- Pratyabhijnahrdayam 2
(By the power of her own will alone,
she unfolds the Universe upon her own screen.)

*J*imutavahana, one who rides the clouds! Parvati, in the embrace of Lord Shiva, being carried above the clouds, was so ecstatic that she gave Him this new name. Kamadeva, the Lord of Desire, the catalyst of all creative processes, whom Shiva had slain, was reborn the moment Parvati embraced Shiva. As the unorthodox hermit, *Ekavratya*, who lived by his own rules apart from traditional society, Shiva yielded to Parvati's soft, sweet words, her smile stirring love in Shiva's austere heart.

The two complemented each other perfectly. She was gentle and divinely graceful; He was wild and forceful. Her subtle *lasya* tempered his energetic *tandava* and created perfect harmony. Together, the Divine cosmic couple captivated the vibrations of the Universe.

Parvati gently enticed Shiva into the ways of the world, and through a myriad questions aroused his concern for the cosmos, Nature, society, life, love and marriage, which He was previously oblivious to.

His great wisdom, acquired through eons of brooding and meditation, was shared for the good of the cosmos. Parvati was the perfect student, Shiva the perfect teacher. Through their cosmic union, the world was enriched by sacred conversations and the secrets of the *Vedas*, the splendours of the *Shastras* and the deep mysteries of the *Tantras* were revealed. Lost in the heights of the summit of Mount Meru, at the very centre of the Universe, Shiva, the supreme yogi and Shakti, his sensual female consort, together view the world. The cosmic couple is satiated with the transcendental peace that follows the ecstasy of their union.

Shiva explained to his consort the meaning of *transcendence*. The whole of existence is consummated in transcendence, which is the goal of all yogas. Transcendence reaches beyond all phenomenal limitations and is the supreme goal of evolution; the ultimate destiny of our creaturely existence. The creative force of Brahma brings all beings into existence, while the preserving force of Vishnu protects their lives. The transcendental force of Shiva leads one beyond worldliness, moving from the mundane to the metaphysical. On the highest level, transcendence is the complete experience of reality beyond both worldliness and death.

Each of these deities is inseparable from its respective counterpart, the feminine energy or *shakti*. In *Tantra*, every higher principle exists through the union of male and female forces. *Shakti* is the essence of sheer bliss. Through *bhakti* or devotion, she uplifts the force of faith. The *shakti* of Brahma, Saraswati, is the patroness of the 64 traditional arts. These arts and sciences add to the charm and eloquence of a person.

Without such modes of expression, our lives would be devoid of zeal, ardour or passion. These arts form a means of communication and self-expression for our deepest urges. Shiva's consort, Kali is the initiator to transcendence. A woman becomes one with Kali by coming to terms with her own awesome power of initiation. Lakshmi, Lord Vishnu's consort, is the pure embodiment of preservation, prosperity and beauty. The triad of the three forces of creativity, transcendence and preservation correspond to birth, death and life in our very existence.

Love unites us to the source, the supreme creative force in the Universe, where Shiva and Shakti merge.

Shambhavi, the State of Seeing Shiva

'Shambhu Sundari, the undecaying immortal form, by the eye of yogic vision I
extract the soma from the crown chakra and offer it to you, who dwell in the
enkindled kundalini fire in the muladhara.'
– Ganapati Muni

My life is where I want it to take me — on a path of love, passion,
ecstasy, healing, peace and calm. Love may not be the deepest
love I truly search for, but I keep working on myself and never for a
moment get disheartened from the hope that one day I will find what
my heart really searches for, and what my fervent prayers seek.
Meanwhile, I am in ecstasy and wake up every morning with a feeling
of being cherished by the Universe.

Shambhavi, the *namakaran,* my spiritual name, reflects the new
energies arising deep within me and flowing out into the cosmic
consciousness. The sound of the letter *'sh'* was what my birth chart
indicated, but my parents had other inclinations. Through recent
searching and deeper delvings into Shiva-Shakti energies, my *chahat,*
the inner quest, for a name relating to Shiva seemed to play in my
heart. As a deep insight during an intentioned meditation, the name
Shambhavi arose in the thoughts of Vamadeva as he searched for a
name of Shiva's consort that was unusual, but profound.

Maybe he too was guided by Shiva's consent, as the Moon was located in *mrigashiras*, the *nakshatra* or constellation, ruled by *soma*, when the name winged its way into his heart. *Mrigashiras* is the head of the slain antelope and also symbolises the head offered to the Divine. When we offer our minds to Shiva, the *soma* flows freely through us. We become one with His consort as Sundari, the *devi*, who manifests the highest beauty of perception.

Chhinnamasta, the Maha Vidya Goddess whose image is a severed head, like this *nakshatra*, represents the consciousness beyond the mind. She makes us cut off our own heads and dissolve our minds into pure awareness, freeing us from the limitations of the mind and its *maya*. When we cut off our heads at a mystic level, it is not blood but *soma* that flows. In this way, Sundari and Chhinnamasta are one.

The source of well-being for the whole world — the state of Shiva called Shambhu — gets expressed as the gaze in *shambhavi mudra*. In this practice, while keeping the eyes half-open externally, one directs one's attention within, this being one of the great secrets of the *Tantras*. It is, as it were, directing one's attention to Shiva and merging the world back into Him, which is the natural movement of *shakti*. Shambhavi is the form of the goddess who represents this process of offering one's eyes, mind and head to Shiva. So Shambhavi is also Chhinnamasta and Sundari, cutting off the outer world of desire but opening up the inner world of *soma* and *ananda* in its place.

There is a strong healing energy in the name and a power to manifest teachings. *Sham* also means *shanti*, peace and indicates the balancing of *prana* and *apana*, Sun and Moon energies, time and space, Shiva and Shakti. Shiva as Shambhu is closely connected to the Himalayas and to Ganga and their healing powers. In addition, *sham* is the *bija*, the seed *mantra* for Shani Deva, the planet Saturn, which grants us enduring peace.

Having no fear of walking in the deep woods, or losing myself, I know there will be someone, somewhere to hold my hand and lead me down the path. I simply place my trust in the Universe, knowing every journey ventured provides an important lesson. Now my heart always sees a reason for the pain that comes my way; it only makes me a more sensitive and compassionate woman. I have learnt to deal with it all and move on.

Listening to the heart makes it easier for me to accept life as it is. Experiences unfold in my life, seducing the mind and taming the senses, always drawing closer to the heart, unveiling deep secrets, hidden anguish, the pain, truth, beauty, sensuality, and joy — the very expression of life! With total surrender, offering myself to the higher powers of the Universe, *sadhana* has transformed my life into a love affair, but a love affair with all that is.

Thus *Tantra* became the essence of my existence, manifesting my spiritual path to enlightenment, teaching me to embrace and unify the erotic and the sacred dimensions of life, all of which are rooted in the spirit. *Tantra* guides us into enjoying the beauty of the five senses in our everyday moments by surrounding ourselves with what we ourselves value as most beautiful, colourful and sacred.

My spiritual awakening altered forever the way in which I perceived and experienced the world. Once that turning point is reached, there is no going back to one's earlier comfortable mindset. Through *Tantra* I cultivated the skills of opening the heart, visualising, focusing, letting go of the mind, being fully present, loving the other and myself, and moving beyond every fear.

Life is about acceptance, moving on. Denial is not what I believe in any more because what one resists will always persist in a subtle form. My life becomes one of passion, but for me passion is pure energy, the fire, and the sheer existence of every aspect of life. If one is praying or meditating without passion, without intensity — without the fire — the deeper unfolding will never happen.

Passion must become the thirst, the very hunger, the connection between you and the greater existence. There is the possibility of one's whole being becoming consumed by the fire of this passion, but to reach beyond mediocrity, we must live a life of intensity, fervour and ardour. This is the real experiential truth about *Tantra*, not the popular stereotype! Sheer passion seemed to be kindling my inner flames, raising the fervour of *agni*. Shambhu is also the blessing of the fire. My passionate sojourn began with Shiva!

> 'Nothing exists that is not Shiva.
> There is nothing apart from Shiva,
> there is nothing other than Shiva.
> To be aware of Shiva is to be
> fearless and free in the self.'

Shiva is Life

'Yatha tatra tathan yatra.'
- Shiva Sutra 3.14
(As here, so elsewhere.)

In the beautiful hamlet of Kanatal, tucked away at 8,000 feet in the Himalayas, spending most of my time in contemplation and meditation, I was blessed with the most beautiful experiences. From the bay windows, which formed two sides of my room, I would look at the magnificent, towering, perfectly shaped branches of the *deodar* trees. Their strong essence would waft into the room through a haze of misty clouds, their vital force nourishing both my body and mind.

The *deodar*, Himalayan cedar, gets its name from the Sanskrit *deva-daru* (divine tree), its timber being used in temples for doors, walls and roofs. There is no denying that the *Deodar* is the noblest and most godlike of trees in its powerful stance, moaning to the strong winds, never bending, the melting snows sliding away from its resilient branches; such is its *rudra* energies.

I spent lazy afternoons lying on grass spotted with wild irises under a haze of the palest shades of pink apple blossoms. The air diffused with the sweetness of their aroma, I drifted off into a wonderland of mystical thoughts to the drone of the flitting bees overhead. The bees brought to mind the trance-creating meditation of the *bhramari* breathing *pranayama*. I wonder if the *rishis* originally learned the secret from the bees.

Nature has been my foremost guru. And I have placed my heart for healing many times at her lotus feet for she is truly *Bhu Devi*, Mother Earth, or *Bhuvaneshvari*, who is Mother Nature personified. Surrendering to Nature one's being that is overcome with the illusions of *maya*, she gently heals and comforts us.

The deep red hues of the rhododendron-flower-bedecked trees against the mountain skyline reminded me of the sacred red colour worn by brides in our Vedic marriage ceremonies. Red, the colour of passion-play, the purity of the flame of *agni*, fire, the depths of the red rose, the sensuality of a red mouth, the magic of the red Sun over the ocean — such were the hues of my love and passion for Shiva.

Trees represent the highest form of consciousness in the plant kingdom, their energies reflecting both the cosmic masculine and feminine powers. In our experiences with Nature, our beings sense these male-female energies; we just need to relate to the innate sensitivities of our hearts. To me the *deodar* always brings out the 'Shiva' qualities as these trees exude more masculine energies, overpowering one with a silent subtlety. On the other hand, the beautiful rhododendron exuded the 'Shakti' quality, the prevalent energy vibrating with Her powerful 'active' force. The blood red hue and texture of the flower give vent to the woman's potent menstrual cycle, the texture of the petals showing the soft, silken sensuality of the female body.

Magical moments seemed to be the essence of my life. We were looking for a statue of Shiva to place in the remote village temple on the hilltop. There were so many alabaster statues of all deities in the shop, and my eyes set upon a statue of Shiva sitting majestically on a mountaintop. Alabaster lends a softness of expression in its form. He seemed to be breathing life.

I guided the artist on how to paint the statue, visualising the colours to be used to adorn Shiva's form. Visualisation helps us focus the energy released through prayer and meditation. The inherent vibrations in the stone can express a powerful spiritual presence manifesting the deity's stillness. Some of the sculptor's passion in chiselling the statue must flow through, sparking the initial life-force.

The *sthapana*, placing of a statue in a temple, is performed with beautiful rituals. This process includes *prana-pratishta*, establishing *prana*, invoking the deity and imbuing one's heart with its energy. The ritual is performed by reciting *mantras* from either the *Vedic* or the *Tantric* sources, and further combined with visualisation of the deity or the light at the heart centre energising the statue with life, love and *prana*. The icon takes in the consciousness of the deity, thus breathing life into it and connecting it with our own deep inner reality.

The villagers carried the icon in a flower-bedecked palanquin followed by devotees in a procession chanting and reciting hymns. At the hilltop the head priest gave us a warm welcome and began the rituals with the sprinkling of *gangajal*, water from the holy river and a shower of flowers. Vedic *mantras* were chanted and a fire offering made with incense and food, ending with the bells tolling and the local children singing hymns of praise.

Sitting in a corner in a meditative mood, taking in the poignancy of the moment, experiencing the chanting, there was a metaphysical transformation unfolding before me, sweeping me into the fold of its powerful vibrations. The sea of people filing past, paying obeisance and making offerings of foodgrains, sweets, flowers, and incense blinded me. There were intense colours manifesting in woven textures of draped saris, shawls, jackets and headgear.

Raising my gaze as if there was a call, I met the glance of a young nubile child-woman. Her large, intensely dark doe-like eyes set in an angelic frame of heavenly beauty seemed to pierce my soul. She weaved her way through the crowd of men and women, not taking her glance away from my eyes even for a moment. She came and stood in front of me, knelt down and touched my feet. She disappeared before I could even react, leaving me in a mesmerised state. Searching her out but in vain, my eyes welled up with tears, not of anguish, but of a certain benevolence.

I was watching Shiva basking in the glow of obeisance of the multitude, surrounded by incense and brightly-coloured dahlia flowers, the hues of purple and sun yellow, fuchsia and alabaster. He surely seemed to be smiling and in my heart rose the beautiful verse from the *Rig Veda*:

'We have drunk the *soma*. We have become immortal.
We have gone to the light and found the gods.
How can the powers of illusion affect us now?
Oh immortal bliss, what can the harmful attitudes of mortals
do to us any more?'

My Lord appeared before me: *Sadasiva*, the immortal, eternal Shiva; the one endowed with the power of knowledge and who bestows His blessings in the form of liberation. His azure blueness was one of scintillating radiance, eyes lowered with a heavy dreamlike presence. His face before me was the light of pure knowledge, which dispels the darkness of ignorance. His hands folded into the shape of a boat, long gently tapering fingers raised to His lips. His dark hair piled high on His head, resplendent in every conceivable breath and then He faded away into oblivion.

'*Masha* Allah!' arose surprisingly from my lips. It was as if experiencing a holy joy, feeling the gentle strains of a tremulous vibration followed by quiet sublimity. That morning I remained with my secret *darshan* close to my heart. I must have been doing something right. Maybe it was the moments of passionate surrender unconsciously through my *sadhana*, or maybe it was just the right time for me to experience the other world. Those days one always existed in another world. Alone within myself, but never ever lonely, this was my choice and every moment of being alone was enjoyable.

Shiva Disappears

'Vismayo yogabhumikah.'
— *Siva Sutra 1.12*
(Yogic realisations are amazing.)

I was sending distant healing energies to a young friend in London, who was gradually fading away from this world due to the collapse of his liver and spleen. Each day would entail a drive to the nearest town to connect through the e-mail or speak with him over the phone. He used to panic when he would know I was going into the Himalayas for my *sadhana*, so one had to touch base with him every day.

One such afternoon, after connecting with him, I discovered a tiny shop hidden away that had a treasure-trove of beautiful old pictures of all the deities. I began pulling out all the pictures, when my heart stopped for a single clear moment. Right in front of my eyes was the same picture of Lord Shiva that I had seen in the village — His hands curved before His lips, holding the cup filled with *halahal vish*, the poison He consumed of *samsara* which threatened to destroy the world.

Samsara is the ensnarement into the web of worldly existence that creates the cycle of birth and death. And Shiva is *neelakantha*, the blue-throated one, who can drink the poison of *samsara*, turning it into nectar.

My entire being began to quiver. Collecting all the pictures and paying for them, I rushed back to my room. I placed Shiva's picture at the altar by my bedside and that night, I sat and prayed and meditated. Surprises never seem to leave me!

The next morning after indulging in some delicious *aloo paranthas* and the red, nutritious rhododendron juice along with a squeeze of lemon, basking in the sun, I seemed to be drawn back to my room. Lighting incense, settling down to meditate, I realised that the picture of Shiva drinking *vish* was missing. Frantically searching, it remains a mystery how the picture disappeared, for no one ever entered my sacred space. The following day dragged me back to the little shop to search out other copies of my beautiful Shiva. Obviously there was a childlike persistence, and so I bought the other two pictures for my collection!

A dazzling display of light filled the dusk horizon and a nip was in the air when I walked up to my room for the evening *sadhana*, surrounded by the heavy incense wafting through the surroundings. The hour of dusk is in a different light altogether, as the sky in the western hemisphere renders itself into blazing hues of tangerine, magenta, and pure red — more a play of passion while the skies on the eastern side play the more subtle, sensuous, gentle tones of blues, aubergines, pinks all fading into a grey.

On one such dusk, Shiva appeared again, against the backdrop of the hues of the eastern skies, in a most remarkable form — fair skinned with auburn hair tinted with gold and a flowing beard. It is amazing how I also came across pictures depicting these very picturisations and colours following my experiences. I never questioned their significance or gave it too much thought.

To Shiva I open up the depths of my heart, sometimes as a child, yet other times as a woman, showing Him my passion, confiding in Him, asking Him for silly favours, sometimes being very, very personal. Some may have been for visits to His abode, others for a clear or an overcast sky shielding me from the heat of a sunny day. There were no rules for me; even taking the liberty of asking Him to change the dates of my oncoming menstrual cycles, and I would pertinently give Him the dates, so that they wouldn't cause me any inconvenience in my travels to the remote Himalayas. The timing was always perfect.

Yes! I was selfish with Him at times. He always humoured me, for whatever reasons. Such is the closeness I learned to share with Him, where I could be completely in the nude, not just in body, but also in the soul. I built this relationship with Him over long periods of time. I am sure a lot has to do with the *anugraha* or blessings from an earlier life. To me it was all about mastering the play of consciousness, *chitshakti vilas*. My quest was to make every moment of my life a sacred celebration, and Shiva was ever so benevolent.

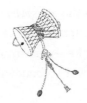

Ananda Tandava, the Celestial Dance

'Nartakatma.'
(The self is the dancer, enacting the states of waking, dreams and deep sleep.)

I related to Shiva as the wild God of eternal power and ecstasy, Nataraja, the cosmic dancer. When Shiva becomes Nataraja, the three primordial principles, the *gunas* of *sattva*-purity, *rajas*-passion, and *tamas*-ignorance, which exist originally in a harmonious, undisturbed balance, are swirled into motion, churning to the energetic vibrations of the *damaru*, His hand drum, shattering the silence of the infinite.

All of Nature dances to the rhythmic beat of creation, ensuing the *lila* or play of the wind with the waves and the tides, the cosmic swirl of the galaxies and the frolic of ethereal beings. From the sound of his *damaru* emanates the primordial sound of *OM*, the first syllable of the ancient Sanskrit language, giving momentum to *akasha*, the ether, reeling forth the other elements of air, fire, water and matter into the motion of life.

Shiva's *ananda tandava*, his joyful, dynamic dance, is symbolic of the totality. The *damaru* represents the continuity of creation, the open hand symbolising preservation, and the hand pointing downwards denoting the destruction of Universe. His foot stamping the dwarf form represents the Universe under the veil of darkness, while His uplifted foot beckons God's grace, *anugraha*.

Why did Shiva find expression in dance and not in sculpting? When an artist completes a work of art, there is a detachment; the two existences separate. One stands back and views the art as an alter ego, revolving around the 'I'. The artist will continue to correct his original strokes, not satisfied with his initial efforts, mirroring himself in the depths of whirling colours and brush strokes.

On the other hand, the dancer loses himself completely to the dance! The dancer and the dance become one; there is unison, a harmony, a reaching into the unfathomable depths of body, mind and soul. No correction based on forethought can be made. The reality of the dance is spontaneous and unpremeditated.

God chose to be a dancer and His dance permeates the omnipresence in every fold of life — the autumnal leaves rustling to the Earth, the subtle hues of the rainbow glistening off the morning dewdrops, the sound of thunder playing the sensuous throbs of the base drummer, and the drama unfolding in the heavens of the twilight zones in a tempestuous canvas of colour.

The interplay of infinite energy and consciousness surpasses all boundaries in the dance of Shiva and Kali, revolving in wild abandonment in the luminescence of the moonlight. Their uninhibited wild union breaks the world asunder, throwing light on the limitlessness of their infinite pairing.

Such is the passion of dance — a beautiful form of meditation, especially if one allows the body to pick up the strains of the rhythmic beat, allowing every drum beat to metamorphose our soul to the heart throb experienced in the mother's womb, bridging one's consciousness of the psyche with the soul. Yet, solo dancing is always more powerful, unless both the partners' energies are fully in tandem.

To be seduced into trance-like ethereal vibrations, one can blindfold oneself with soft silk, creating a certain void or an enchanting atmosphere through the wafting of incense to music dimmed to the glimmer of scented candles and allowing a timelessness to overshadow one's being, elevating the soul to subtler vibrational levels, and giving expression to the self.

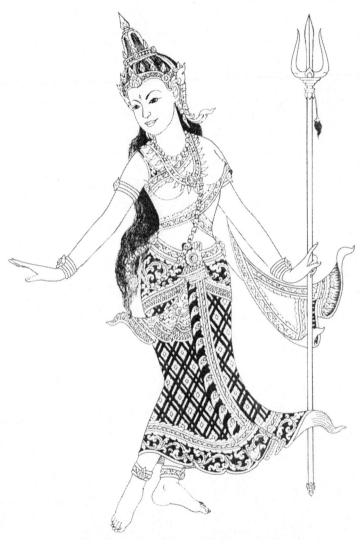

Shakti Sadhana Creates My
Sacred Space

Sadhana is Worship

'*Jab lagi jiyoon daya phal paoon, tumhro yash mein sada sunaoon.*'
- *Durga Chalisa: 39*
(O Ma! Bestow upon me your grace as long as I live, so that I can
always recount the feats of your glory to all.)

Shakti sadhana is the spiritual discipline that leads an aspirant to the realisation of *shakti*, the Divine force within. *Sadhana* is worship and reflects the spirit of love through which we awaken the gods and goddesses within. An expression of one's creativity and attitude is the seed of worship, and *svabhava,* the ultimate ecstasy, is the fruit this *sadhana* bears. Worship connects us to spirituality, regardless of what name or form it takes.

The body, with its solar and lunar energies, five elements, senses and the mind becomes the perfect temple for this inner worship. Through our bodies we are able to commune with our deeper inner self. For an *aghori*, not only the body but also the entire world becomes the temple and the playground for spiritual practices.

Sadhana is the yogic discipline followed to unfold the inner truth, the self or *devata*, a process of learning to discriminate one's thoughts and ego-perceptions from one's true nature. It helps us absorb the nuances of the deity's personality into our subtle body, the astral body. The mind and its thoughts inhabit the subtle body. *Karmas* projected from the causal body must first pass through the subtle body before reaching the physical body for their expression. Understanding these expressions and harnessing them for meditation, helps us evolve to higher levels.

Tantric worship occurs at three levels — internal, external and a combining of both. *Tantra* weaves together the inner and outer realities through all forms of devotional worship — *puja*, the offering of *mantras*, flowers, incense, scents, music, lights and food, honouring the goddesses. But these offerings must be performed with awareness, recognising that the outer form is truly a reflection of the deity power residing within our hearts. Ritual worship helps to channel one's deeper energies. Yet when a rite is performed without knowledge of its symbolism, its metaphysical quality remains hidden and inactive.

The force or beautiful form of Shakti can only reside in a sacred space. She cherishes being idolised with rituals, flowers, incense, sweetmeats, a lit lamp, *mantras* and her esoteric geometric forms, the *yantras*. The sacred space becomes her little corner, though she is all-pervasive, and as much as we enjoy a beautiful space, breathing air and light, so does she.

Shakti is the lightning that pervades space. The lightning or electrical force of pure consciousness pervades the sacred space, allowing it to manifest its various forms of delight. Wherever space is given, Shakti must arise. Space, much like the womb or the Earth or the quiet mind, has a power to create, which arises from receptivity. That is the origin of Shakti, not any effort to manipulate or control.

In most of our homes we only give the darkest little room for this sacred space, sometimes with no windows, restricting the play of the cosmic elements of space, fire and light. The goddess nourishes the vibrations of this space brought about by meditation and *mantras* and the exuberance of *bhakti bhava*. *Bhakti* is the state of intense devotional love creating the *bhava* or emotion, the feeling of absorption and complete identification with God. *Brahmabhava* is identifying with the all-pervasive reality, feeling one with all.

My bedroom became my sacred space, the playground, for my experiences with the higher powers. From a simple altar emerged a most beautiful storehouse of pictures, objects, stones, flowers, aromas and textiles, each taking in the energy of the deities, infused by my passionate prayers and obeisance with the very deep vibrational forces of the *devis*.

The entire power of their vibrations began to permeate my bedroom, my sanctum sanctorum, where I spent several hours cocooned and protected from the ravages of the world outside and my mind within. To worship and deeply invoke the *devatas*, we must create our own sacred space to allow us to retreat at any hour we wish to connect to them. We must remove ourselves from all external factors of time and space, to enter into their *mythic time* and *space* and discover our real inner peace and quiet.

Never embarrassed at displaying my ardent passion for my spiritual beliefs, on the walls were placed beautiful etchings in deep terracotta ink of the great *siddhas* and saints including Ramana Maharshi, Ramakrishna Paramahamsa, Mahavatar Babaji and Sri Aurobindo. My wonderful friend MK specially made the beautiful drawings, translating the treasures of the soul. To me these drawings were never lifeless objects. Unbelievably alive, their eyes pierced the inner soul.

Mahavatar Babaji's piercing gaze moving on one side; Ramana Maharshi's smile following me from every conceivable angle, and the passion for Ma Kali caught in the soulful gaze of Ramakrishna Paramhamsa; whilst Aurobindo reflected a soft, compassionate calm look. There seemed to be a cosmic light emanating as life through their watchful gazes of me, pervading every moment. I felt safe and happiness prevailed around me, in spite of the outer persistent forces of anguish.

Call it narcissistic, but I have beautiful pictures of myself in this sacred space, including a truly intense moment lost in the depths of Divine passion, taken during a moment of meditative bliss on the banks of the Ganga. My spiritual teacher from Bangalore described the picture as 'Shakti emanating from Shiva in a moment of sublime bliss.' Another is a charcoal drawing of me made by a young artist in his twenties, who came my way through my friend, Nani. Sitting in front of me, in half an hour, he captured my expressions through his charcoal lines. He wouldn't allow me a preview until he asked if he could add something to the drawing. He was warned not to take it away from my actual personality.

He gave the drawing its finishing flourishes with what he personified as Ma Durga — her hands in the background and a large *tilak*, the red vermillion mark, on my forehead of the married Indian woman. I was quite taken aback by the drawing, for he had captured the softness yet silent strength of a woman who had experienced the myriad hues of life, with passion, pain, deep anguish and a zest for living life!

The One Reality

'Citih svatantra visvasiddhihetuh.'
- Pratyabhijnahrdayam 1
(Citi creates the Universe of her own free will.)

Our ancient *rishis* teach us that there is one reality, but this true God has many faces and personalities, and each is an aspect of the formless godhead. Each face of God is a deity playing a very specific role in the great cosmic drama. All external forms of divinity are superimpositions on our inner divinity of the soul.

Ultimately, when all these superimpositions have served their need to raise our vibrational levels, all the gods merge back into their own true nature, the one and indivisible Brahman, and then only that reality remains. The *devata* is Brahman, the soul is Brahman and the truth is Brahman. After all eventualities, the entire Universe is Brahman, and all varied paths, however diversified in thought, rituals and worship, must go to this as their final goal.

As we develop in experience, our conception of the *devata* undergoes many changes. Actually the *devatas* never change for Brahman remains the same. It is essentially we who change and how the *devata* appears to us changes accordingly. What we see in our mind's eye is our reality. If we fill our mind with soap operas and acts of violence, then these become our reality, but if we view the *devata* there, then he will become our reality. It is our choice that we see and which is real for us.

The unity of the microcosm and macrocosm explains that

everything that exists in this external Universe, the macrocosm, also appears in the internal cosmos of the human body, the microcosm. The human being is a living replica of the entire Universe, and every figment of the Universe is as alive as every cell in our bodies. The *Vedanta* explains that all the deities are personifications of Brahman created by the soul itself.

The representation of an idol, the metal or stone that gives it shape and identity, is just a medium of expression, carrying within it infinite vibrations that have evolved over millions of years of its natural existence. The powerful *prana pratistha*, life-infusing *mantras*, are ways in which the worshipper connects to the Creator through the representation. It is not of the utmost importance what we believe in or what one's belief manifests as an object of worship. Pure simple *astha*, belief, is what counts, for this belief is the core of our existence.

I have a collection of rocks, stones and wood of varying hues, shapes and sizes, which, taken from all around the world, speak to me of the vibrations of their origin. A shimmering rock with mica sparkling through its surface, smoothened over by time, inscribed with two intertwined serpents from Kedarnath, sits alongside the *Shivalinga* and the *salagram* at my altar. To me everything on the Mother Earth vibrates with a life-force, a collective form of universal energy.

The more time is spent in this particular space to meditate or pray, the more peaceful and potent vibrations will certainly permeate the being. I would often retreat into this space for calm and peace, for the experience of being centred in myself. It created a psychic field of grace for me. I learned to create my own simple rituals, based on studying the objective I wanted to reach, and practiced them in my sacred space.

All forms of devotional worship and *puja* — the lighting of the lamp, incense, offering flowers, or the use of food as *prasada* are useful ways of honouring the *devatas*. They should be performed with awareness and knowledge, realising that the outer form is merely a reflection of the goddess's power that resides within each of us.

There is a scientific approach to *puja* or rituals. Rituals empower our personal space, deepening our connection to the Divine in ordinary life. Through *puja* we spiritually energise the material objects being offered, which helps us connect our outer physical reality with our inner, divine reality. The specific offerings to the deity are significant in propitiating the five elements, as in the use of a nutritive oil for the Earth element; flowers for ether; incense for air; a flame, as of a *ghee* lamp for fire; and liquid food as in milk or *Gangajal* for water.

Truly, I followed my heart in every way. For me there were no rules ever, for every rule in the book has been broken by me. Though I always sought guidance from Shiva, He never put any strictures or conditions in my way. He allowed me to open my heart and soar on the wings of fiery passion into the wilderness of His Universe, experiencing joy and tumultuousness, bringing me back to the reality of suffering and pain, each time putting me through the grind of His tests, so that my *sadhana* would deepen.

Anjali, an Offering to the Divine

'The only offering that truly enriches is the one that is made to the Divine.'

Amidst the vibrational energies of the Himalayas, in the meadows of Kedarnath, the flickering eternal flame within my heart would allow me to transcend all bodily limitations and find unabounding deep serenity, surrendering myself and making an offering of my soul at the lotus feet of Lord Kedar. Through *bhakti* or sheer devotion, the essence of light would expand, pervading the surroundings and baring the depths of my soul to the healing balm of the Earth's vibrations, with the flow of Shakti, the Goddess of Energy, in the form of the sacred waters of the River Mandakini. Creation seemed to reflect itself as a timeless presence in these dwellings, speaking of the endless Divine manifestations.

Ancient cultures are revered for the beauty and depth of their customs and traditions. Our Indian culture with its ancient traditions is steeped in scientific, logical, mythological, social and spiritual significance. Understanding this depth lends meaning to an otherwise mundane procedure of customs and superstitions. The tribals of remote India and the Pueblo natives of America preserve the sanctity of Nature, making offerings to the Mother Earth in deep gratitude, giving back what they have manifested from her for their livelihood. They kindle their souls in fire, air, Earth, water and ether and are still at home in the non-human world.

Agnihotra or fire worship is a simple Vedic form; *homa*, an offering of our inner fire to the universal fire. The worship of fire is powerful in its ability to neutralise negative forces as well as to heighten the positive forces within us. *Agni* is literally fire as a transformative force and is symbolically associated with heat, energy, austerity, asceticism and illumination. It is the fire within each of us, which on being awakened through *sadhana* directs the ascension of the *kundalini*.

We offer to the fire *ghee*, rice grains, special woods from particular trees, cow-dung, sweets, condiments, and fragrances, which convey their subtle essences to the deity. Fire has the power to conduct and magnify our thoughts and wishes for peace and prosperity. The same fire, setting us free from negativity, can consume negative emotions such as anger, hatred and fear. Sesame oil and pure *ghee* lit in lamps are both nutritive and *sattvic* in nature, nourishing the subtle form of the *devata*, sustaining its contact with our physical existence.

Trataka or steady gazing at a source of light, particularly *ghee* lamps as a yogic technique, helps us focus on the outer light in order to develop the 'inner light' within our hearts. It is a form of meditation in which one stares fixedly at an object and if done properly, can open the third eye. On a physical level, it helps improve the eyesight and concentration. The eyes bring us the gift of light, our sight that nurtures our inner faculties of perception and imagination, creating beauty around us. The beauty of Nature prevailing in her diverse forms as trees, blossoms, the wild grasses, flowing rivers, or snow-capped mountains, all stimulate higher intuitive powers and elevate the soul through the spirit.

There are three primary forms of *trataka* practice. The *inner trataka sadhana* consists of closing the eyes and focusing the attention on the point in the middle of the forehead, the location of the third eye. It helps in building deep concentration and higher levels of patience and

Anjali, an Offering to the Divine

intelligence, removing all negative thoughts. It raises the intuitive levels in a person.

The *middle trataka sadhana* focuses the eyes on a flame kept at a distance of 20 inches at eye level. This improves eyesight, concentration, memory and mental power, relaxing the mind and increasing one's working efficiency. The *outer trataka sadhana* can be performed at any time and any place, simply by focusing one's attention on any object one sees, like the early rising Sun, the Moon or the stars. It also improves one's eyesight and concentration levels. Gazing at the Moon is very beneficial for the eyesight and calms the body, mind and soul.

However, though, those suffering from heart ailments and eye diseases should be cautious in practicing *trataka*, particularly using bright light sources.

Our sense of smell relates to inspiration. Fragrances and aromas uplift our spirits creating the mood to experience transcendence. The use of different incenses invokes different *rasas,* awakening and energising with mint and *patchouli*; opening the heart with rose and *bergamot*; expanding the spirit with sandalwood and lavender or creating a sensuous mood with jasmine and *ylang ylang*.

Incense allows us to unravel our deepest experiences. It is purifying and soothing, and most importantly, helps us commune with the 'other world'. The goddesses, deities, spirit world, angels, our ancestors — all feed on incense. It is the most profound way of paying our obeisance to them, an offering of the inner subtleties to the higher echelons!

The offering of something sweet to the Divine beings holds immense symbolism. The sweet offered takes in the vibrations that we generate whilst praying, chanting or meditating. When we consume it as *prasada,* these same vibrations will be absorbed deep into every tissue and cell of our bodies, creating a gradual transformation in the consciousness of the *sadhaka*. As a practice, I would leave raisins overnight in a tiny silver server and have it as *prasada* whenever I needed to energise my being.

The flowing Ganga cascades from the locks of Lord Shiva, all rivers being forms of the Divine Mother, since water is the female energy in creation. The goddess's benevolence, beauty and bounty flow forth from these rivers as her blessings. In our homes in India, we always have some sacred water placed in a copper or silver vessel, used to purify and energise the home with its sprinkles.

The *kalasha*, a metal or clay pot, is filled with sacred water, with five mango leaves decorated at its mouth and a coconut placed on top. This *kalasha* represents the inert body which, when filled with divine life-force, sustains the power to manifest all our wishes. The water in the *kalasha* symbolises the primordial water energy from which the cosmos and the entire creation evolves.

The first offering of water is made at the break of dawn as a salutation to the rising Sun. Then an offering is made to the *tulsi*, holy basil plant, in the form of the *tulsi matham*, an altar bearing a *tulsi* plant. In Sanskrit the *tulsi* is incomparable in its qualities, *tulanaa naasti athaiva tulsi*. This sacred plant symbolises Goddess Lakshmi, the consort of Lord Vishnu.

Flowers in Offering

'Flowers lift towards the sky their fragrant prayers and aspirations.'
—The Mother

Each flower symbolises an aspiration, an emanation, and a Divine quality. A flower radiates beauty, joy and tenderness, a sweet aroma to all that surrounds it. The Indian woman always adorns her hair with flowers. Beauty is the joyous offering of Nature. Flowers symbolise the deep connection between the cosmos and our psychic world. They absorb the negativity, pain, stress, and excessive heat from our beings and release it, giving us peace and happiness.

Flowers find expression through silence, stillness and beauty. This is because their means of expression is less developed than that of the human being, but their soul still has a voice. They are truly a manifestation of the psychic in the plant world. Forming a deep love and conscious contact with flowers will make us receptive to our higher self and awaken us to our psychic or heart consciousness.

I became aware of the consciousness in plants and their intense aspiration to live, spending time in Nature among the trees and plants during my *sadhana*. Plants need sunlight to live; their whole lives are truly a worship of light, a light that contains divinity. The Sun represents the supreme consciousness. Plants aspire intensely to catch the rays of sunlight and will make every effort to reach out to it for their survival.

This is their consciousness; their very will to live! They will find a way to touch the strains of sunlight, even at the cost of mangling their shapes.

The blossoming of every flower reflects the dynamism of the Divine feminine, which encourages growth with an affirmation of the promise of bounty. I wonderfully applied this metaphor to my own *sadhana*. During *sadhanas* in the night, at times I experienced an intense burning heat arise that was intolerable. I would have to remove my clothes, dampened as they were with sweat. To cool the body I learned to use flowers, wonderfully wrapping my naked being in strands of marigold, red roses or *mogra* flowers. Amazingly, the heat would come up to my neck but then suddenly dissipate, leaving my body soft and cool, drowned in a realm of subtle and sensuous aromas.

During the Navaratri, my room would be filled with red roses; the petals strewn all over and which were lovingly brought from a farm by my driver Sanjay. In every nook and corner of my home, there would be roses floating in shallow bowls of water. The consciousness of both the pristine water and sensitivity of flowers took me beyond the boundaries of my senses into a poetic mystical realm.

Flowers are very receptive and rejoice in being cherished. To be receptive is to experience the urge to give and the joy of giving, the ultimate gift being an offering to the Divine. It is through the aura of flowers that Nature expresses herself most harmoniously, bringing out her inner soul.

Each *devata* has a special fragrance that it prefers, defined by its own lineage, power, colour or aroma. The Himalayan lotus, the *brahm kamal*, is used in the worship of Shiva by Shaivites, its boat-shaped, waxen white petals sheltering a dense cluster of purple flower-heads. The red hibiscus is pure beauty that exists for the Divine and by the Divine. The flower is a consecration of the goddess's Divine grace; a gift the Divine gives us when we unite ourselves with her. The purity of the lily is an apt offering to the Madonna.

Worship of the planets is an important form of spiritual rejuvenation. Flower offerings to appease the *nava graha*, the nine planets, are made as per their characteristics and inherent nature. Red flowers to the Sun, Mars and *Ketu*; white flowers to the Moon; yellow flowers, the marigold to Jupiter; white fragrant flowers, the jasmine to Venus; violets to Saturn and *Rahu*; green leaves to Mercury.

The *Vamachara tantras* interpret flowers and incense for their inherent potency in an intrinsic way. The *pushpa* or flower is referred to in the context of the menstrual flow of blood in the woman in the *Mahakala Samhita*, classified according to the age and aspects of the Shakti. Through *mantra, tantra* and *yantra* and other *Tantric* rituals, the worshipper carves a sensuous and sacred niche from out-of-the-ordinary reality, paving the way for ecstasy.

The lotus flower in *Tantra* symbolises the different *chakras* in the human body, each petal denoting a *bija* or seed *mantra*, opening up the inner magic. As our energies open, flow and swirl within us, they create vortexes like flowers. Our soul is such a flower in space.

Flower Petals in Healing

*'Santa dyauh santa prthivi santam idam urvantariksam
santa udanvatir apo Santa nas santvosadhih.'*
- Atharva Veda, 19.9.1
(Peaceful be the heavens, may the Earth be calm, and the spacious
atmosphere gentle. May the flowing waters, rich in moisture, be
soothing; may all the plants and herbs be beneficial to us!)

Flowers remind us of the sweetness of the power of surrender to the Divine. There's a deep silence expressed in their sweetness, often more revealing and expressive than words. Plants find expression in sheer silence and beauty, raising towards the sky their fragrant prayer and aspiration. Flowers stimulate our senses, inviting an emotional response to their colour, fragrance and beauty. The strong sweet aroma of the wild rose evokes a sensual mood; a field of lavender lifts our spirits instantaneously. The emotional response, that the inherent quality of the flower brings out from us, forms the basis for healing through flower essences.

Flowers are beautiful symbols of love and act as healers in their own diverse ways. The healing energy of flowers can be distilled with spring water and charged with sunlight or moonlight. Medicines or tinctures are prepared from this mother essence. Remedial flower essences help balance the disharmonies in our deeper mindsets. Our bodies manifest diseases as a result of imbalances in our emotional and spiritual make-up. Floral essences work on these emotional imbalances, healing the body, mind and soul in a gentle manner.

The offering of flower petals or garlands in rituals and ceremonies is a global custom. It is also a form of emotional and psychic healing.

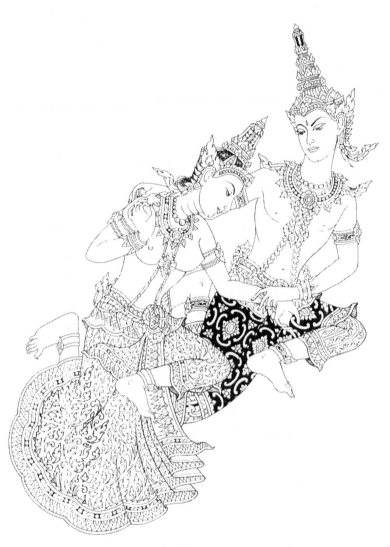

Bhakti Yoga:
The Strains of Love

Bhakti Unfolds Adoration and Ardour

'Om parama prema rupaya namaha.'
(*Om* and salutations to the supreme form of love!)

The path of *bhakti yoga* was my choice for *sadhana*. *Bhakti* means faith, devotion, dedication, adoration, and ardour. These attributes rendered the impossible possible for me. On my spiritual path, faith dissolved any self-doubt, while devotion hastened the realisation of my goals. The devotional love that manifests from Radha's absolute consecration alone has the power to bring down Krishna's light into the mind and heart.

Faith can best be explained as a deep feeling of knowing and believing; there can be no questioning. The yoga of devotion was my form of communion with the deities through ritual worship, visualisation of the deity, *mantra japa* and meditation. My heart was constantly seeking a connection with the Immortal Power.

Supreme love is the highest yoga. *Bhakti* is devotion and like Christian and Sufi mystics, the yogi cherishes the concept of love as the simplest means of reaching out to God. The path of love involves no penances, asceticism or painful tortures of the body, yet the act of surrendering one's ego and worldly desires is not easy. Radha and the *gopis* of Vrindavan merged completely with Lord Krishna, freeing themselves from worldly jealousies. Their dance, *raaslila*, remains one of the highest celebrations on the path of love.

Each seeker's route is his or her own as an individual. Traversing our own particular path, our temperaments and experiences give shape to its uniqueness, bringing about a subtle culmination of *bhakti* with *jnana*, knowledge, touched by our *karmas*, tempered with *seva*, and the practice of various techniques. The incidents were numerous which guided me to find my way to seek divinity — ecstatic moments, chance meetings, death, accidents, misfortune, a thought, a sudden effulgence of Divine grace — one never knows from where the call will be heard.

In the *Srimad Bhagvatam*, Krishna says: "Many are the means described for the attainment of the highest goal...but of all, love is the highest; love and devotion that make one forget everything else; love that unites the devotee and me...as all earthly pleasures fade into nothingness." The path of love is considered supreme because it is wholly selfless. The Universe was created for love and that love is the very purpose of our existence. It confers *ananda* and softens the grind of a mundane existence.

Sufi literature and music are rich with the raptures of devotional love. *Bhakti* unfolds as a transcendental experience of bliss, a mystical surrender through a passionate yearning for God, rendering Sufism in its essence as timeless. Sufi mystical poetry is a synthesis of thought, feeling and imagination and ardent passion, which awakens deep inner senses giving expression to the mystic spirit. Sufi music would transform me into the realms of divine *nasha*, a state of drunkenness in my meditative moods to the soulful renderings of Nusrat Fateh Ali Khan Saab and Begum Abida Parveen.

For a while I shied away from being in love, having been deeply hurt, till it dawned on me life wouldn't be a pilgrimage without the anguish and pain wrought by love. Accepting that love will always bring a certain pain, but knowing the possibility of reaching higher levels of consciousness through this pain, my creativity touched its zenith when wrought with agony and ecstasy. We may want to experience ecstasy without going through the pain of loving, but one has to experience the dark night to be able to set sight on the rising Sun and bask in its first gentle rays.

I learned not to despair from the experience of a relationship that had not borne any fruit because there is every possibility of intense love rising out of it anyway. Somehow love worked as a ladder, guiding me to attain higher levels of compassion. After all, it could start with one person and find succour with all beings in the form of human kindness. Because of the selfish attitude that arises out of attachment, sometimes the control factor is the root cause for love becoming painful.

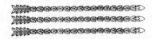

Raino follows her Heart

'To be wounded by your own understanding of love;
and to bleed willingly and joyfully. '
- Kahlil Gibran

My beautiful friend Raino brought home this deeper understand ing through her experience with love that began over the internet. She was vulnerable, having spent considerable time in meditation, being happy with her lot in life. Breezing into her life with an e-mail id scribbled on the corner ripped off from a page, her friend Sheena played a dramatic role in introducing her to a man named Shokha.

Trusting in the play of the Universe, Raino got drawn in with the words he had typed out in his e-mails, never for a moment doubting the sensitivities of the man behind them. Till one day she realised e-mails were being exchanged with Sheena as well, inviting her for a rendezvous at a far off island. Hurt set in, but her purity of heart caused her to still trust him anyway.

Shokha her new beau, who had the experience of several years behind him and had a shadowy view of life and women. A few months into this banter over e-mails, Raino gathered her savings and flew out to the Garmisch area in Germany to meet him. She was frightened, but we all gathered around her to provide her support in this adventure.

Little did we realise this would be an adventure to say the least, leaving her dealing with some anguish and deep bruises over the following months. She meditated all through her connecting flight, praying for everything to work out well. His magnetic presence was there at the airport and trembling, she took the rose from his hand, and seemed to melt into his gentle embrace, shyness enveloping her being.

The ethereal beauty of Nature seemed to calm her nerves and she surrendered to love, making her world go round, waking up to a beautiful morning, the Sun playing hide and seek after a brief drizzle from the clouds above. Then her witty remark pressed a button somewhere inside him, giving rise to deep resentment. Suddenly his lover -boy demeanour disappeared and out poured angry hurtful words from him, revealing some inner pain. She was left stunned, until her calm nature came to her rescue. Shokha drove off and Raino decided to take refuge in Nature's embrace. Tears rolled down her cheeks, giving rent to gentle sobs, half way tempted to pack her bags and fly back home.

Nature's soothing balm seemed to heal her heart and she decided to stay on for the entire duration that they had planned. Mood swings played to the winds of a deep distrust in the Universe. And there were tender moments too, understanding glances and warm embraces. At times Raino's calm demeanour seemed to send ripples into Shokha's universe.

Sometimes we grow up without ever realising the true strains of love. Life seems to be a battlefield of power, money, ego, control and distrust, which becomes an alter ego in the due course of time. All love must begin with oneself, be it the physical self, emotional self or mental self.

Maybe some day Shokha would realise that he toyed with the sensitive heart of a woman bearing the subtlest vibrations. Sometimes one has to become like the fool in the Tarot deck in order to experience the reality of truth. In experiencing these follies we gain a certain wisdom of moving on and letting go. One can never build one's own happiness on another's pain; eventually, the price of this pain will be levelled out.

The purity and sanctity of love must be honoured. Raino's deep pain absorbed itself into the strains of Acker Bilk's beautiful song, *"I'll get along, and you'll find another…"* Pain has a sweet way of reminding us that Divine love is the purest love, in spite of everything! His memory lingered on in its own gentle way. Keats simply put it, 'Beauty is truth and truth is beauty'. The highest form of beauty is not on the outside but on the inside, for external beauty can only reflect for a moment a greater internal beauty, which transcends all forms.

Some people have a set belief that physical attraction is the beginning and the end of love and they miss out on the opportunity to evolve. Others abstain from a physical relationship as they neither recognise it as the beginning nor the end, so lose out on a beautiful experience, with eventually their pent up frustrations disturbing them at another level. Yet some know that the right physical chemistry is the beginning, not the end and develop it as a means of experiencing higher levels of consciousness. The idea of pure love must be nurtured through sensitivity and care.

Kshama, Forgiveness

'Om dukha hantrayei namaha.'
(*Om* and salutations to she, who eradicates the sorrows of this world.)

In spite of my own personal experiences of disillusionment in rela
tionships, I learned to expect much happiness from the future by
remaining in close contact with cosmic consciousness, not allowing
anything to stand in the way of a meaningful and happy life. I came to
understand that worry never improves one's circumstances, yet also
realised how difficult it can be to let go of worry. Conversations and
arguments between people seemed futile and take up a lot of energy.
How can one rationalise another person's actions? How can one
understand another's mindset?

Dealing with my own mindset seemed an easier way out of such
situations. I searched out the cause for the pain within, which almost
always lay deep-rooted in the psyche. There was never any use in
blaming the surrounding world. At least I had the power and
intelligence to change myself. My prayers and the Divine powers always
showed me the light. Accepting it gracefully, no matter how painful it
was at that present moment, I always moved on to happier times.

Learning to detach from negative situations and persons, I used
various forms of meditation, visualisation and affirmations. And most
importantly, I forgave my own follies and those of the other,
understanding the *karmic* unfolding of our lives. Looking at oneself
deeply is a continuous path for self-growth. Along with the honesty of
understanding one's own mistakes, we must also learn to be gentle

with ourselves, loving and nurturing the heart and soul within. The more one fails in life, the more one needs to love and be gentle with one's self.

Viewing the larger picture, seeing the destruction, hatred, intrigue and conflict in the world, one must understand that nothing is truly negative. Negativity has a distinct function within God's creation. Negativities shake us out of our self-imposed peaceful existence, exposing the play of *maya*, which creates a false sense of self-contentment. The dark forces are part of the illusory duality and can never be completely eliminated. Yet one must ask, 'How then must we deal with this devious dark force and its effects manifesting in anger, hatred, cruelty and violence?'

Kshama, forgiveness, supremely harmonises our inner soul with the cosmic consciousness. Forgiveness doesn't translate as an approval of negative actions; it gives us the choice to free ourselves from reactions to them. The inability to forgive holds us to negativity, binding us to past actions. Acts of violence, traumatic experiences, or infidelity, whether in this lifetime or carried forward from another, make it difficult to forgive. These are imbedded in the subconscious mind, keeping the negative experiences alive.

Freeing ourselves from this bondage is possible only by facing the situation and being willing to forgive, not by judging the cause or the reason. There is no explanation for good or evil as both have their purposes at particular times. Ultimately, through Divine love one is able to truly forgive, not finding reason in the deed, but understanding that the person is seeking satisfaction in external circumstances. For those living in Divine consciousness, the emotions of hate and revenge are irrelevant.

To forgive is truly divine because it takes courage to set aside what is often a very justifiable anger. But when we make this choice and allow ourselves to forgive, we actually do ourselves a great service as this allows us to let go of pain. It is easy to become attached to seeing oneself as a victim and holding on to this resentment. Forgiving is one of the most difficult and most spiritually rewarding choices that we can make for true healing in our lives to occur. When we are ready to release anger and to forgive, it will always help us internally, whether or not we intend to express these intentions to the person who has hurt us. It doesn't matter if we aren't in touch with the person any more.

Just concentrate in your mind's eye on the person you wish to forgive, without dwelling on their past hurtful actions or words. Sincerely wish everything good for them that you would want for yourself, be it happiness, worldly comforts, good health or peaceful times. Repeat this concentration for as long and for as many times as it takes before you sense a positive change flowing from and to your heart. It may be a period of days or weeks before you really sense this. You will surely realise the positive shift of freeing yourself from anger and pain.

Forgiveness is not just a noble act; research definitely shows that the person forgiving benefits as much, perhaps even more than the one who is forgiven. Expressing true forgiveness empowers one because it helps us to stop feeling like a victim and dispels our own suffering at having been wronged. Our levels of anger and hostility diminish while our capacity to love increases. Our trust and faith in people is restored.

Through compassion one becomes detached from the power of negativity. Hating, cursing or surrendering to their forces only enhances their energies. The victory is in neither being seduced nor intimidated by their disturbed actions.

I found a way through Vipassana to bring about equanimity and equipoise, and to create an inner awareness. Self-realisation comes through experiencing the satisfaction of accepting one's lot in life through wisdom and knowledge.

Kshama, Forgiveness

Mudra, Spiritual Power Forms

Ritual gestures or *mudras* express the inexpressible through their contours, awakening and communicating with the deities or higher energies within. The *mudra* is a mystic positioning of the hands, forming certain yogic symbols and culminating in finger power points co-related to specific organs in the body or areas of the brain. These gestures aid in concentration and channel energy through their shape and structure.

Mudras have a wondrous effect on our emotional being, our feelings and moods, healing the deeper levels of the soul. These hand exercises stimulate the brain, and when done with concentration and in a serene state, our cerebral activity is calmed and regenerated. The simple exercise of running one's thumb along the fingertips in a gentle and conscious way can feel wonderful, calming the brain.

Atmanjali mudra or the gesture of prayer activates and harmonises the left and right sides of the brain. To do this yourself, place both your hands in front of your heart *chakra*, leaving a slight hollow space between the two palms, in a comfortable position, while you are either standing or sitting. This gesture supports deep inner collection, creating balance, repose and peace. Try to experience the energy rising within you, through your hands, bringing the inner self to silence.

Shivalinga mudra is an energy-charging *mudra* that removes depression, dissatisfaction and tiredness, bringing about an inner healing in the body and mind. To perform this, place your right hand, with the thumb extended upward, on top of the left hand, which is shaped like a shallow bowl. Hold the fingers of your left hand close together. Position your hands at the level of your navel, elbows pointing outward and slightly forward. Stay in this position for four or five minutes, at least twice a day. Sit in a comfortable position, relaxing the breath during the process. This position balances the *yin* and *yang* energies.

Sublimity in Love

'It is not the 'presence' of someone that brings 'meaning' to our life,
but the way that 'someone' touches our heart, which gives life a
beautiful 'meaning'.'

As we mature in devotion, our experiences of longing deepen and eroticism is experienced in relation to the world of the Divine. Love is the nourishment of the soul, a prayer that can lead one to the Divine. Love is an expression of gratitude, thankfulness, and celebration for no reason at all; it is an unraveling of the mysteries between man and woman and all of life. Love heals, comforts, renews, inspires and empowers us to walk to great heights; all real love is based on the search for the inner spirit.

When they conjoin in a holistic consciousness, man and woman reach beyond the mere physical cravings of their sexuality. Creating a spiritually intimate energy field of love and prayer, they 'raise' themselves in love. Our individual uniqueness can only be experienced through the divinity of love. Without the deep inner fulfilment of love, people will be influenced by the illusions of physical attributes, fear, insecurity and envy, experiencing temporary gratification that ultimately ends in a void of discontent.

Experiencing Divine love and compassion, we perceive the spiritual power of unconditional love. This awareness brings about a sublimity and calmness into our existence, making us aware of the temporary nature of all physical beauty and material things. We release ourselves from the threat of duality, past and future, seeking comfort in the presence of eternal love. In this sanctified harmony, man and woman will experience a connection to the higher forces of consciousness, bringing about love and integrity between themselves and in their families.

Loving Commitment

'But let there be spaces in your togetherness, and let
the winds of the heavens dance between you.'
- Kahlil Gibran

The bond of true commitment holds a couple together, creating absolute trust. When committed to another, one experiences truthfulness with one's inner self as well. Sharing the truth with the beloved, we create a sacred space to overcome life's turbulences. Loving commitment, whether formal or informal, provides a deeper meaning to the relationship. Encouraging the couple to share their innermost feelings and release any past guilt allowing them to experience the joyous sharing of love. Opening up your heart to another by expressing your deeper feelings leads to a mystic bond of trust.

Making love is a beautiful opportunity for establishing a lasting bond of commitment, and when there is the motivation of true love, a couple is ready to explore inner sexual secrets. In *Tantric* teachings, a wish made in the heights of ecstasy will unfold into a reality, unifying the couple and taking them to exalted states of higher dimensions of love.

Love is the ultimate nature of the Universe. When we are deprived of it, our bodies and minds suffer, raising our blood pressure, restricting our breathing, even sometimes causing heart failures. Lovers in long-term relationships can pour into each other's fold the wealth of sheer joy, fulfilment, passion and ardour. The sublimity of love can shower untold blessings upon us! But for this we must be steady in holding the love within us.

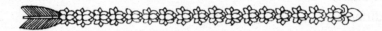

Irresistible Desire

'Love has no other desire but to fulfil itself.
But if you love and must needs have desires,
let these be your desires.'
- Kahlil Gibran

Irresistible desire can be a manifestation of love, a release of emotions expressing the physicality of love. The beauty and wisdom of *Tantra* guides us to embrace sexuality as the doorway to one's 'ecstatic' mind of great inner bliss. The yoga of sexual union leads to an enjoyment of all the powers of the senses, enriching our being with deeper *rasas*, accessing the flow of *shakti* along the path of liberation. In *Tantric* idealism, desire must be understood in order to experience all aspects of a deeper, higher love. Sexuality is an integral part of human nature, which, when approached with reverence, can translate into altruistic energies, taking the individual to higher spiritual levels.

It is an act of reverence to regard the body as a temple, creating awareness in its physical and subtle cosmic fields. Keeping the body beautiful, pure, healthy and harmonious is a way to connect to the divinity within. By worshipping in the temple of our body, love is magical, raising levels of energy and fulfilling deep desires. In the act of lovemaking, we should unfold the body into an altar of joy and bliss. *Tantric* love leads one to an ultimate experience of cosmic ecstasy, through awareness of the higher inner self in both the partners, unfolding all aspects of emotions and intellect.

A split between the heart and the head can create immense psychic disunity, causing a dysfunction of intimacy in the relationship, in the long run leading to sexual disorders. Most ailments are psychosomatic, resulting from negative thought waves. A deep distrust in the Universe and in oneself creates an inability to love. Frequent experimentation with different partners actually can create a 'performance' fear leading to sexual dysfunction. The use of aphrodisiac drugs can create a temporary sustaining factor but results in an even deeper fear of poor performance, resulting in deep-seated agitation and anger.

Negative sexual habits in the long run dull the senses. A sexual encounter or pleasure without love or feeling can damage a person's psyche. Self-examination can help us on the evolutionary path of love by turning our consciousness inwards to reflect with honesty our hidden psychic impediments. Examining the inner self can resolve and strengthen our mental attitudes, bringing about a state of clarity, helping us eliminate the negative emotions that cloud our relationships.

Relationships where there is a lack of emotional fulfilment result in unresolved *karmas*, creating resentment and deep anger. Understanding the play of *karma* in our relationships will throw light on the erratic events that result in relationship failures.

During lovemaking the vital forces of the two individuals blend, bringing about an interchange in their *karmas*. This exchange affects both their individual and joint destinies. The nature of this interchange depends upon the degree of consciousness of both persons involved. If loving compassion is the intention of the consummation, a positive *karmic* exchange is created.

Tantric love rites should be attempted only with someone you truly love; not used as an experiment to hopefully create more pleasure. In ancient times, masters raised their own as well as their partner's levels to higher states of consciousness through *sadhana*. Today, such a deeper orientation is very rare; making lovemaking a mere physical act. Many *Tantric* teachers lead people astray, emphasising unusual actions over any inner feelings. Making love with a stranger during *Tantric* practices,

Irresistible Desire

which they sometimes recommend, is usually more damaging than elevating to the psyche of a person.

Most relationships go wrong, without both partners understanding the real cause. The couple should observe, share and discuss their relationship failures before moving on, if they don't want to repeat the same mistakes in the future. Dealing with the issues of failure brings about an acceptance at a deeper level, initiating the real healing process. By working out their desires consciously, both people can learn to master their own destiny, embarking on a more positive and fulfilling journey into the future.

We all cherish having someone as a witness to the unfolding of our lives, viewing the highs and lows, the love and anguish, reaching out to our weary souls and raising a toast to the sunshine!

Children of Life's Longing for Itself

'For their souls dwell in the house of tomorrow,
which you cannot visit, not even in your dreams.'
— Kahlil Gibran

Driving from New Orleans to Natchez for a vacation with friends, I was overawed by the ponderous effect some of the trees along the way had on me. The live oaks covered in Spanish moss were tall with grey-like drapes. To me they seemed surreal. Natchez has an old world charm about it. I spent wistful moments at Kathryn and Edward Killelea's 'Clifton View' home serenely situated on a cliff-top overlooking the Mississippi. I sensed powerful undercurrents of male energies flowing in the river.

One early morning, spending time with Edward's nieces (little angels they were), in the setting of their garden, amidst us was the most serene statue of Our Lady, who seemed to interact with us, showering her blessings on us in that early morning hour and creating a magical spell. I held the children spellbound, travelling into another world, spinning stories to them about my existence as a Red Indian squaw, riding bareback on wild white horses through the wilderness, sleeping under starlit skies, making conversations with the trees, flowers and bees. The little girls were losing themselves to the wonder of my stories, when overwhelmed with excitement, they ran inside to narrate to their grandfather the stories of my escapades.

We can learn so much from being with children and their open minds, free from the burden of knowledge and experience. Their childlike exuberance takes in the innocence of the wilderness. Chasing butterflies from an unknown world; they unfold an abundance of love, purity, trust and happiness. This happiness is a meditation of the soul, looking within our 'inner self', the touchstone of innocence.

Ishana, my younger son, brought close to my heart the prayer of gratitude, for God and His grace came in the form of love. Having lost his hearing to the confines of silence, he grew up to be a blessing, bringing to me the awareness of the finer nuances of *karma*. He grew up into a young man with a stoic inner silence and a great sense of humour.

All our revered *siddhas* living in close tandem with Nature had their divine experiences in its fold. The inner world is far more extraordinary than the outer world. I learned to delve inside this 'inner world' and experience bliss. No matter what man chases and acquires in his waking state, at the end of the day he retires weary eyed. He may acquire wealth, laurels, and power but at the end of his waking hours, it is *Shramraj*, the Lord of Weariness and Tiredness, who welcomes him into his arms.

The heart centre is a medley of deep emotions, thoughts, knowledge, desire, love, joy, lust, and anger. Called *anahatam*, "unstruck", this *chakra* or psycho-energy centre is the seat of extra-sensory perception, higher intuitive perception and intelligence. We need to enter and discover the magic of the 'heart centre' — delve into its hidden treasures, deal with its passions and idiosyncrasies and heal the self with its potions of magical balm. Life is a phenomenon of its energy.

Touch is usually a physical experience, but there is a different kind of touch that is not necessarily physical. The real touch, the meditative touch, is the healing energy flowing through Nature, permeating the Universe. The person who consciously chooses to be receptive to this touch gets healed. A meditative person may not physically touch a person, but his presence becomes a healing source, comforting the soul for anyone who happens to be present in their energy field. Saints remain alive for eons, their energies permeating not just their tombs, but the trees, birds and animals in their surroundings. This is the reason some of us still experience their vibrations at their tombs or temples.

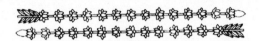

Anugraha, in the Wake of Blessings

'*Evam vidham gurum dhyatva jnanam utpadyate svayam
tatsadgurupraasadena mukto hamiti bhavayet.*'
— *Gurugita 98*
(By meditating on the guru, one gains knowledge spontaneously.
By the grace of the *sadguru,* become aware; 'I am liberated'.)

When all doubts and experiences born of time are burnt to sameness with the fire of consciousness, the yogi enters into the state of grace, and the true self is revealed to him. This is called *anugraha.*

Divine grace is unconditional. It is the free and supreme will of Goddess Shakti to bless a *sadhaka* who has evolved beyond the taints of the ego. It is the *bindu,* the point between anywhere and everywhere, and cannot be obtained by any mere human effort. Grace may descend upon anyone, whoever it chooses, at any time and any place. It is beyond the human intellect to understand the play of grace, which is spontaneous and uncalculated. Only the deserving *sadhaka,* aware of divinity, may arise to the occasion.

In my life, the way of *shaktipat,* grace, benediction or compassion found itself unfolding through Nature's blessings, endowed with the reverberations of Shakti. It transformed my being, consuming all impurities and awakening the inner self, dwelling in each of us, the supreme guru.

Nature created the abundance of *kamadhenu*, the wish-fulfilling cow, bringing life to fruition. In Nature, I found both Shiva and Shakti in different aspects of the same tree as its firm roots and flowering beauty, exuding a beauty of aromas and auras. The rivers of the Himalayas release their *shakti*, energy, into their flow, undulating and winding their way around the steadfast boulders, speaking a silent language of eons gone by. Each strong shower of rain brings down with it numerous blessings in its very expression of fury.

My early understanding of *anugraha* and *shaktipat* came from teachings of Baba Muktananda, a great guru and spiritual master of a few decades ago. He had initiated my *sadhaka* friend, Mahajanji, in 1968 and through his renderings of experiences with this guru, I came to understand the play of *shakti* within us that opens up our minds to higher experiences which are directing us to Divine consciousness.

As Baba Muktananda gently brought to mind, God hid the key to heaven in a place where people couldn't find it: in the human heart. Baba called this key *shaktipat*, referring to the Divine energy that a *siddha* guru can at will bless upon a seeker, awakening his inner consciousness to realise God within us. The Divine energy released within is known as *kundalini shakti*, the beneficent goddess, who is lying asleep within us at the base of our spine. Once the *kundalini* is awakened, she begins to move upwards through the seeker, purifying the entire being on physical and subtle levels leading us to experience the Divine sweetness that is in each of us.

The guru is the visible form of *Parabrahman*, the all-pervading Brahman taking the form of the Universe, and it is this that enters into the *sadhaka* in the form of grace. The activating of this grace is called *shaktipat*, initiation, the true *kriya yoga* or guru's grace. The grace is the infusion of *rudrashakti* into the *sadhaka*. This grace stays with the *sadhaka* from birth to birth, no matter where he is re-born; his spiritual *karmas* eventually bear their fruit, activating the grace.

Deep faith in the manifestations of the Divine grace takes us beyond the need to comprehend its action in our lives. No one can understand the extent of the *anugraha*, the Divine grace behind everything, which organises everything in our lives for us to move forward to the Divine realisation as swiftly and harmoniously as possible, adjusting the prevailing circumstances around us.

Once this grace is bestowed upon us, there is no conceivable point in time or space that does not connect us to its miraculous ongoing work, the constant flow of grace in the Universe. Witnessing this grace, we should never have any fear, anguish or regret, or even suffering. Living in tandem with grace, our life becomes the sheer exultation of infinite happiness. For each one of us it is the path that leads fastest to the lotus feet of the Divine.

My experience with the Divine, be it through my visions during *sadhana* or in deeper restful hours, brought this *anugraha*, creating a surge of intoxication, unending plays of light, voices, metaphorical messages, celestial sounds, overwhelming ecstasy, and the flow of immense happiness making the most ordinary things seem beautiful and abundant.

Mantra japa brought its own energies into my life. Some of these were bestowed on me through realised souls, others guided to me through visions or specific thought processes. The *mantra* must be deeply imbibed as the form of a higher worship, with complete faith and sincerity, allowing its *rasa* to flow through our being, absorbing it into the *prana* or life-force behind the mind. Meditation is an infallible means of conquering the restlessness of the mind, the master key to opening up the inner knowledge taking us gently down the stream of love and abundance.

I deeply searched out the eternal guru in my life, a man who had been through the intense fires of *sadhana* himself, knowing the force of *agni*, its innate power to burn as well as its healing energies — a man in touch with the subtle *rasas* that exist in Nature, taking me gently into his magical fold, bringing to fruition the innate *shakti*, energies residing in my being. Meanwhile, I work with Shiva's *shakti*, hoping one day He will guide me to experience my deeper self in tandem with His choice.

I used to question the love of mystics with sheer curiosity. What

I used to question the love of mystics with sheer curiosity. What must their state of euphoria be like? Was it like the all-consuming passion that is experienced by lovers? Only till I began to experience a similar euphoria welling up inside me, waves of love and ecstasy, joy and sweetness in the sheer bliss of meditation, did I find my answers in the depths of silence.

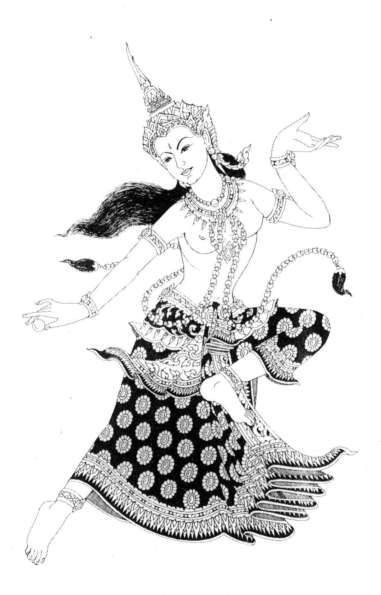

Tantric Rhythms of the Cosmos

Tantra Connects Me with the Universe

'Svecchaya svabbittau visam unmilayati.'
—*Pratyabhijnabrdayam* 2
(By the power of her own will alone, she unfolds the Universe
upon her own screen.)

The essence of *Tantra*, which means a fabric, is 'connectivity'— connectivity of the inner self to the vastness of the Universe, to the very subtleties prevalent in the cosmic energies. It requires changing the range of one's vibrations to pulsate alongside with the higher vibrational levels of the cosmos, delving deeply with the macro and slipping gently into the micro orbits of forces.

When we lose contact with the natural world, our fundamental roots get shaken, disturbing our relationship to life and Nature. Our concrete, busy city lives disconnect us from the magnetic healing powers emanating from the Earth. But when we spend time with Nature, particularly with an open mind and heart, we can harmonise with her rhythms and energies.

Tantra is the science of the human form, its body, mind and soul. We simply need to align our human form with the prevailing cosmic energies. To me the prevailing cosmic energies are to be experienced in the presence of Nature, where we learn to listen to the rhythm of the cosmic forces. Nature is the primal, original sacred space, which nourishes and cherishes us through Mother Earth. Nature heals us emotionally, spiritually and physically, revealing our true godhead that breathes life into every miniscule atom that wills its energy to enter into form.

We are caught up with proving and disapproving subjects on science, religion, money, people, or countries, spending our energies in the controversies of everyday life. We wake up to a life of newspapers, radios and televisions — all formats of borrowed knowledge, borrowed incidents. We allow ourselves to be dragged down into this vast fishnet that traps us in its fine mesh of other people's news and gossip. We forget how to swim the beautiful waters of the inner ocean, the sheer experience of the wave as it rides a high, forms a crest and breaks with the even tide, rushing to the shores.

Our day begins with second-hand experiences and we carry these vibrations of connectivity to our brain centres throughout the day. Is this the existence we were born to experience? Is this the life we choose to live? Is this the world we want to share with future generations? We need to begin making changes right away, this very moment, if we want to really live, see, feel and be aware of the great totality of life.

Scientifically, *Tantra* has been experienced and documented by our ancient seers and *rishis*. Yet today it is mainly only a matter for brilliant books that remain sitting on shelves in bookstores; sometimes it is denigrated to mere sexual antics.

We need to bring the spirit of *Tantra* into our everyday lives and begin living it from moment to moment. A point comes when we have to leave logic and rationality behind and just listen to Nature for a while, discerning her subtle inner voice, and receive the ultimate understanding, not in the ordinary sense of mental knowledge but in the mystic sense of direct feeling! Logic is clearly man-made. Even if we insist on being logical or rationale, existence is not going to change according to our logic; rather our logic must interpret this change to understand true existence. I simply made my choice to live life as a mystic.

And I began worshipping Mother Earth through her powerful manifestation of Nature. Through Nature we will purify and pacify our body and mind and thus reach the deeper levels of our soul, which is true divinity. With Nature, we have to feel it, understand its vibrations, appreciate its hues, and learn to know it, for there is no way of expressing it except through direct contact. Experience is the golden key, the master key that will open the locks of all the mysterious ways of Nature.

Spanda, the Universal Resonance

'Sabda brahmeti yacchedam sastram.'
(The scriptures say that sound is Brahman.)

Spanda, its omnipotence resonates in its various meanings: a throb, a vibration, trembling, an explosion, movements, an arising, or expansion, a reflection, or the ultimate unfolding! *Spanda Karika*, based on the experiences of the *siddhas*, consists of 51 verses that unfold the principles concealed in the *Shiva Sutras*, forming one of the most important treatises of Kashmir Shaivism.

Modern physics explains matter as waves of differing lengths, without the presence of anything essentially solid, what can be called vibrations in our layman's language. The *Trika Shastra* conceived centuries ago called it *spanda*. *Tantric* Shaivism explains the entire matrix of energy pulsation of which physical reality is only one part. *Spanda* is the energy that permeates the Universe during its process of evolution, a ceaseless force from which all existence evolves. *Spanda* is the supreme universal *shakti* through which all manifestations of ecstasy, joy, sorrow, anguish and pain, the complete spectrum of emotions is embodied through the impetus of spirit. It is the dynamic aspect of transcendental reality.

Abhinavagupta, an important exponent of Kashmir Shaivism, observed *spanda* as unobjectified desire, which leads consciousness to experience its incompleteness, thus being the first stage of awareness before crystallising into the reasoning process. Through introspection, an aspirant can experience this inner motive force of *spanda*. Ramakantha, the author of a commentary on the *Spanda Karika*, has explained it as an inner rhythm of aesthetic spiritual experience, which can be characterised as a flash of thought or an inner perception such as pleasure or pain. *Spanda* becomes the first flutter of pure consciousness in the process of its five primary actions: emanation, existence, dissolution, concealment and bestowal of grace.

Prevalent in the Universe are both forces of good and evil, manifesting in each one of us. We can connect with the subtler vibrations of superconscious levels and begin improving our lives by surrounding ourselves with positive, healthy-minded people and with Nature and all her beauty.

I have experienced such connectivity with Nature's *spanda* on varying levels of its intensities; the gentle *spanda* of the flowing currents of the water, which carry healing vibrations, the mood of their flow weaving its own story into our lives. The vibrations of a tree will vary in its different forms, with usually the older trees carrying more intense vibrations. Placing one's hands on the tree's trunk, one will experience gentle currents passing into the body as subtle vibrations emanating from the soul of the solitary flower in the wilderness.

Nature Shows Me the Light

'Sanno vatah parvata sannas tapatu suryah
Sannah kanikradad devah parjanyo abhivarstu.'
- Yajur Veda, 36.10
(May the winds blow pleasantly for us, may the sunshine shine
warmly on the atmosphere, may lightning shine and roar for us,
may the clouds waft us with graceful rain.)

The art of 'connecting' and 'surrendering' will come to us when we reach out through both 'heart and soul'. Everything carries its vibration. We need to realise and develop these vibrations, which will guide us to connect with our inner selves. Nature is the simplest, purest and surest tool to guide us to realise the self. One must rise from the macro levels of enjoyment and realisation to the micro levels, from the gross to the subtler experiences. Totally identifying oneself with Nature is in itself a state of 'no mind', a state of deep meditation, a state of connectivity.

Step out into Nature and experience the subtler self, the energies and auras of the trees, the exuberance of the breeze, the fragrance of the flowers. Feel the softness of the dewdrops under your bare feet, attune yourself to the buzzing sound of the bees and open your arms wide and embrace Mother Earth. Surely she will manifest in each one of us the beauty and gentleness, the balm and healing of her powerful magic!

In ancient Greece, the Earth was personified as Goddess Gaia, our point of connection with the entire Universe, the source, which nurtures us all. Scientists today use the same term for the coherence of our global ecosystem and its fragile ecological balance; we should all be responsible residents of this Earth. In India, the Earth is worshipped as the sacred cow through *bhoomi puja*, expressing the same reality.

Holidaying once in Goa, taking in the sunshine and the volatile sea, I became very aware in myself of a certain deep curiosity for the unknown. I was in my 30s at the time, brimming over with a wild and zestful curiosity for life's explanations and searching out deeper questions. Then I saw, holding itself majestically in the centre of the courtyard was a very old tree, unique in itself.

The tree had a perfect shape: its branches shading the hearth around it, stoically silent. Its only aspect of wildness was the deepest shades of tangy peach colour blossoms dressing one particular portion of its fold, the rest being densely green leaves. This was the expression of its mood and character. I would draw the energies of this great tree into my being and experience a powerful sensation permeating my body. It resembled a soft sensual embrace.

Trees fascinate me, everywhere in the world, as I realise they were my first silent gurus, Nature's sentries, standing tall! Their intense vibrations filtered through me, calming me, their energies healing my being, sending waves of sensation through me, stilling my thoughts and sending me into a spin of deep questioning. I grew to relate very personally to the vibrations of trees. There were times they would draw me into their fold magnetically.

During a visit to Santa Fe, New Mexico, some years ago, the very vibrations of the Earth played magic on me. Standing in isolation was this tall tree, making a lonely statement. It would actually beckon me into its vicinity. I woke at dawn to step outside in the cold and watch its play with the first rays of the morning Sun. In deep sleep I visualised a *nag* and *nagin* (male and female cobra) meeting in its shadow. This tree had an immensely magical effect on me, taking me into its mesmerising spell on several occasions. As a result of this, I captured some sensitive shots of it at sunset and sunrise with my camera.

Nature Shows Me the Light

Wish-fulfilling Stones

'Even as the stone of the fruit must break,
that its heart may stand in the sun,
so must you know pain.'
- Kahlil Gibran

Stones have always drawn me to their inert nature, their varying hues and, above all, their deeper silence. Stones surely carry their own inherent vibrations, sometimes of the place they represent, but also of the people who have been around them. Using stones for healing, wish fulfilling, or seeking guidance has been a part of my experiences with *sadhana*, seeking the soul within the stone.

A stone-attracting spell can be used for *Tantric* purposes with any stone you feel affinity with, empowering it in your left hand, which serves to gather energy. Visualise energy pouring out from your body into the stone. Gradually you will feel the power increasing in the stone. Charging the stone with your inner wish —be it for love, spiritual connectivity or worldly needs — the stone will create gentle vibrations in order to fulfil it. With the prayer, 'So be it, thy will be done', place the stone in flowing water. Once it contacts the currents of the water, the process of manifestation for your wish will begin.

My most revered master shared with me his beautiful experience of energising stones with *mantras*, so that the stone chants the *mantra* through the water that flows over it. It created magic for me. *Lingas* and *salagrams* can be used as such *mantric* stones as well. All stones are composed of crystals, which resemble very minute *yantras*. *Yantra* is the form and *mantra* is its vibration. This is true in the mineral kingdom as well.

Similarly, to rid oneself of unhealthy habits, hurtful feelings or disturbing emotions, visualise a part of you as entering into the stone. When you sense its vibrations in you, release the stone into the water and flow with its grace. I have the most beautiful collection of stones and rocks from all over the world, sharing with me their deeper secrets of time and events.

'*Om shrim shriyei namaha.*

(Salutations to the creative abundance that is the very form of this Universe.)

Geopathic Stress Causes Tremors

'And since you are a breath in God's sphere, and a leaf in God's forest,
you too should rest in reason and not move in passion.'
– Kahlil Gibran

The imbalances in our environment caused by concrete construction, landfill sites, burial grounds, underground cavities, mineral concentrations or the felling of trees causes the Earth a lot of stress. The earth has its own ways of expressing its 'geopathic stress'; it could be through natural disasters or by just emitting negative energy or producing poor yields in vegetation and crops.

Our ancient culture paid deep reverence to Mother Earth and understood the importance of protecting her energies by offering regular prayers and constructing medicine wheels. Nature worship is prevalent among tribals to this day. They live in tandem with the universal vibrations, and hence are sensitive in apprehending natural disasters.

We need to neutralise these sensitive areas of stress on the planet by being more environment-friendly, preserving Nature's abundance, planting more trees, conserving the mountains, resisting the use of pesticides, encouraging organic farming, and protecting our wildlife. We need to give back to Mother Earth with gratitude what we keep depriving her of.

Driving through the Himalayas for my *sadhana*, a deep fear takes over my being at how people are so insensitively raping the innocence of these sacred mountains, leaving her threadbare through the felling of trees, slicing away her sides to give rise to high rise buildings, destroying her innocence by playing with mindsets of the local inhabitants, putting a price on their heads and buying out their livelihood in the form of land. Today the very existence of the Earth is being threatened by the negative forces; there is an urgent need for all of us on Earth to work and pray collectively to the Supreme Soul for protection and the healing of our world.

Quite simply, we must mentally understand that the play of the Universe is not enough. Every day someone arrives with a new theory and we spend all our energies figuring out its workings. We find less and less time to experience the simplicity of living life in the presence of the moment, forgetting to experience the little joys that carry us into the deeper realms of bliss.

Each of us is a special being, walking one's own chosen path. In this journey, we unveil deep secrets, ecstasy, hidden anguish, pain, truth, beauty, joy, and passion, yet we should not forget to experience the precious miracles of everyday life!

The Stars Reach Out from Heaven

'Om tare tuttare ture sarva shantim kuru svaha.'
(*Om* and salutations to Tara who is the source of all blessings,
please bring peace to all.)

I grew up as a child believing that the celestials are truly from the stars, and as a woman ripened for life, I experienced Tara, in her *ugra*, fierce form. Maybe it seemed the time of maturation, the time to make my offering to the higher powers had come.

Ma humoured me with a downpour of nearly one hundred meteors, in the balmy night sky of a waning August Moon. I was aware of the phenomenon to take place and coerced my gentle friend Daddo to drive me out of Delhi into the wilderness of a farmland expanse, literally luring him with the promise of steaming coffee and *gulab jamuns*, the indulgent Indian sweetmeats.

We drove out in silence at the midnight hour, a deep excitement stirring within my *muladhara chakra*; these were earthly desires, having yet to raise them to a higher *chakra*. Arriving at the open expanse, we were ushered into deep darkness with the electricity failing. To me it was the heavens preparing for a starry fiesta, never failing to pick up the signals. A cool breeze began to lift from the warm hearth, as if answering a silent prayer.

I lay down on a *taktha*, an expanse of wooden planks resting on four legs, calming my being with the *japa* of my *rudraksha* beads. The child is forever within us, when my arm cut through the piercing silence of the night, with an exclamation of joy, pointing to a falling star. The crescendo of naive exuberance rendered me breathless as my eyes darted in all directions taking in the wonders of cosmic energies at play.

The Universe can play an operatic wonder of sound and light, a spectacular performance of great magicians unfolding their cosmic magic! Between 2 a.m. to 4 a.m., I counted eighty-six shooting stars; between the two souls living the wondrous moments Daddo and I reached a count of over a hundred meteors. The rush of adrenalin drew to a close and the skies cast heavy shadows of approaching dark clouds, when from literally nowhere I sighted fierce flames of fire, lighting up the dark dawn sky with a luminous golden glow in contrasting hints of citric.

We stood fixed to the Earth in sheer awe of the dancing flames, when thrusting itself from the middle of this fire was the exhilarating luminescent, the waning sliver of *Chandra*, the Moon Lord! Our hushed silence found an exuberant coherence of expression and from the depths of my heart came forth praise for *soma*, the sweet nectar.

'Om som somaya namah Om!'

The Moon is not only a physical body composed of particles; it is the life-giving Mother Energy, the creative force, which is magnetic and positive. This energy affects our imaginative, reflective, intuitive and subconscious being, granting us sensitivity and sentimentality. The Moon reflects sunlight through its alchemical reflector made up of luminescent crystals. These crystals filter the sunrays, enhancing their hues of light, creating a medicinal effect on our planet. This explains why medicinal plants are more potent during the night under the direct glow of the moonlight.

Tara means a star and is derived from the root *tri*, meaning 'to scatter', as I had witnessed the stars being scattered in the vastness of the heavens. Ma always seemed to shower Her blessings upon me with abundance, filling my life with more zest and childlike curiosity about Her higher realms. Gentle drops of rain began to cool my face and bare arms, raising my energies to the *heart chakra* and warming my being with a softness of love and blessings.

We drew gently out of the daze, beginning our drive back home in the wee hours of the morning. Perched right in front of us were three magnificent wild owls, their eyes glinting in the beams of the headlights. My heart searched for the three goddesses in their presence or was it Tripura Sundari!

Getting off the beaten track on to the main highway were two magnificent elephants leading the way. Unmistakably to my heart arose the thought of Lord Ganapati removing the obstacles, seemingly so many at times. The test never seems to end; on the path, everything is a challenge. I tried to flow with the rough tide and ride the waves with sheer abandonment!

My revered master brought home to me the powerful role of Ma Tara as the high priestess, the chief judge among the *devis*, and Tara, the saviour, who takes us across the ocean of turbulences. She is the star of our heart's aspirations, the beautiful muse who guides us along our creative paths. In my seeking of protection, I turned to the *Tara sarvanga kavacha mantra*, seeking help from Tara for all aspects of my being. Durga and Tara are often seen as one, though Ma Durga represents more the power that destroys one's obstacles and difficulties and Tara, the power, that ferries us beyond them. Tara guides us to rise to higher echelons of self-realisation.

Ganga Flows through Rishikesh

'Swagatam Gange, sharanagata Gange, subha swagatam Gange.'
(We welcome you Mother Ganga, we take refuge in your holy waters,
we seek the shelter of your Divine grace.)

Mine has long been a deep love affair with Ma Ganga, the river of faith bursting forth from its icy womb at Gangotri, flowing from the very heart of the Himalayas. The Ganga is beautiful, almost caressing and nurturing in her nature, arousing deep love, a sanctity and respect in the people who commune with her. The Ganga seems to offer mankind everything through her gentle, yet powerful disposition, the deep glens and forests, the vast expanses of open valleys graced with an abundance of cultivation in tiers of terraced fields forming patterns of yellow, green, burgundy and gold.

I would meditate for hours in her deep flowing icy waters, subtly aware of each wave and ripple, watching butterflies flit around, feeling their gentle energies as they would come and perch themselves on my naked shoulders. The river taught me complete surrender, making me experience every little energy shift within myself. It brought about newer revelations of perfect harmony in solitude, enriching my life.

Her sacred currents unravel the stream of life's energies, the flow of mankind's wisdom, reconnecting death with the stream of life. The magical *soma*, the divine nectar offering, poured over the *Shivalingam* undulates in her waves of Shiva's *shakti*, energy. One grows accustomed to the flow of the Ganga, undulating and calm on the surface at most times, yet deep and powerful beneath.

Having spent time by the rivers in the Uttaranchal vicinity of the Himalayas, I understood that even the rivers have their own nature, moods and particular handwriting. Descending from Kedareshwara, the Mandakini is so sensuously divine; her movements one of tumultuous passion in some areas, yet gentle and smooth in others, taking the boulders with a bit of mirth in her stride, a childlike exuberance of wanting to meet up with River Alakhananda at Rudraprayag. Yet River Alakhananda flowing from Badrinathji is more masculine in her flow. There is a sense of being trapped between the boulders, thrusting forth with a different temperament; even her colour takes on the hues of the Earth, ripping away the soil from its embankments.

During my traverses to the mighty yet serene Ganga, I began to feel the pulsating vibrations and beautiful energies in the stones strewn around. There were stones in the shapes of the *Shivalingam*, with the sacred markings of the *tripunda*, heart-shaped stones, in varying hues and sizes including a three-dimensional shaped heart. My son would set about looking for one for himself, deeming it unfair at not having found a heart, despite his being at the tender age for love.

It was all about timing; each heart stone brought with it a deep secret and in its wake a silent healing. The duality of the magical quality of stone is revealed in that as it is both the generator of life and as the phallus it pierces the woman's virginity perpetuating life, while as the dealer of death it is used as a weapon of war and hunting.

Nadi stuti, which means 'in praise of the rivers', is an important hymn in the *Rigveda*, the 5,000-years-old religious text of Hinduism. The *rishis* always loved and lauded the great Himalayan rivers. The Ganga represents both the river of life and death, for every Hindu wishes to have his ashes after cremation cast into its holy waters. The *namavali* or the various names with which devotees invoke the Ganga has 108 appellations ranging from, 'Thou who were born from the lotus feet of Lord Vishnu'.

The Ganga is revered both as a goddess and as a mother, drawing into her fold innumerable millions who bathe, offer prayers, and drink her holy waters, freeing the soul of past *karmas*. She is the nectar of life and a source of deep inspiration to all her *sadhakas*. The Ganga symbolises ancient Indian culture and civilisation, flowing 2,500 kilometres from its source at Gaumukh, an ice-cave at the foot of the Gangotri glacier (which in recent times has receded some 18 kilometres due to global warming).

Once, while on a plane flight to Varanasi, I started chatting with a lady from New Mexico, sharing my views about the common vibrations in New Mexico and the Himalayas. There was a sense of magic in New Mexico, with an awesome timeless dimension prevailing. I'd relate to the trees and sunsets emblazoning the sky, lifting my spirit into its gentle embrace and creating meditative nuances in my inner consciousness.

The lady gently tapped my arm as if to bring me back into the present moment. Opening her bag, she took out a pouch filled with little folded pieces of paper. Curiously enquiring about these little notes she explained how all her friends, relatives and co-workers had written all their anguishes, pain, hopes and wishes in these little folded notes requesting her to immerse them into the holy waters of the Ganga.

They too were aware of the power and magic of Ma Ganga. It brought me back to my experiences that manifested in her flowing waters. She understood the human heart and soul and had absorbed all my pain, sorrow and deep anguish.

During my second Vipassana meditation, I met Novella, a sprightly young Italian girl, who had spent six months in Rishikesh. She came to stay with me and we both drove down for my 38th birthday. This stay humbled me in several ways. We lived in the Parmartha Ashram, rather spartanly — no worldly comforts, eating in the tiny local *chai dabbas*. Breakfast was rusks dipped in tea, sometimes having to share the next table with my driver Sanjay, who, embarrassed, would get up and leave.

Breakfast by the river became a ritual of wonderment. Each morning between sips of hot tea, we would watch a flowing white-bearded *sadhu* pick up a litter of newborn puppies and carry them into the sunshine from the cold shadows of the huge rocks under which they were sheltering. The mother would patiently follow him to and fro and eventually settle down to nestling her pups. Such an endearing sight! May Ma Ganga always shower her blessings on him!

We made a ritual of feeding the cows and every day we would step out with *rotis*, leavened bread, or bananas. The cows began to recognise us and would converge towards us, gently feeding from our hands, at times nudging us from the back to draw attention. The shopkeepers were quite amused. In India, we worship the cow, for she is *sattva*, pure, the quality of love and light, and mentally very intelligent and serene. She is the perfect mother passionately devoted to her calf and caretaker. If her calf dies, the cow refuses to give milk.

Having grown up on a farm in the small state of Nabha, in the Punjab, we closely watched my mother relate to these animals lovingly. I learned through experiences the behaviour patterns of cows and buffaloes, the cows being extremely gentle in nature with a deep motherly instinct. The reason we try and consume only cow's milk or *ghee* during intense *sadhana* is due to this *sattvic* quality inherent in them and their products.

There was one amazing couple with gentle souls: the husband was blind and the wife would take care of him. One would hear him singing beautiful *bhajans*, spiritual songs to the accompaniment of the harmonium, as they sat happily through the cold winter months and sweltering summers alike, with always a smile upon their lips. Every day we would take them *chai* and rusks. It has been 10 years since I have been regularly spending time with them on every visit to Rishikesh. The quaint town of ancient *rishis* was a bedlam of experiences, vibrations, divinity and divine people.

In a secluded alcove near the cave of a hermit popularly called Baba Mastram, wading into the aquamarine crystal waters of the Ganga, one could experience that although deep and swift, the river never loses its serenity. Being a number two numerologically, water seems to draw me into its whirlpool. The sands beneath my feet seemed to give way and I felt myself drawn inwards into the depths of a tumultuous swirl; a strange, powerful feeling gripped me, bordering on slight fear.

Drawing myself consciously out from this whirlpool, I reached for a rock nearby and clambered onto the white sands. I lay on the sand, allowing my being to take in the cosmic energies that were playing strange games with me, till the energy seemed to flow back into my legs, enabling me to get to my feet.

The Silence of Ramana Maharshi

'Who am I? Who am I? Who am I?'

The Ganga *arati* at the Parmartha Ashram brought many a deep emotion to the surface. The wide alabaster steps leading down to the Ganga where Shiva sat magnificently, basking in the glow of the setting Sun, the crescendo of *mantra* chanting, the fire of the *homa* and serpent *arti* stands casting glints into the vibrant air. In a rapturous moment against the flaming colours of an evening Sun, there appeared before me the face of Bhagwan Ramana Maharshi, his fiery eyes emanating a deep gentle glow, searching the depths of my soul. Silence seemed to blank out all other sounds and his silence began to speak beyond words. I wonder if I ever understood the magnitude of his message; his *darshan* seemed to suffice, and at that moment it simply spelt magic in my life.

Rishikumars, from the tender age of five to young adult men, dressed in hues of saffron with turmeric and sandalwood paste markings across their foreheads, were milling down the stairs to take their place near the flowing Ganga. In their midst would alight the gentle slender Swamiji, endearingly called Muniji, whose beautiful voice would send forth deep love through the strains of the *bhajans* in tribute to Ma Ganga.

During my stay at the *ashram* a call was received by a gentle voice asking to meet me, saying, "Swami Veda Bharati here." Taken aback, we decided to meet at his *ashram* the following day. There was an old charm about the place, solitude, and beautiful vibrations, chirping of birds from the branches of trees having weathered several storms. One had read his books of discourses on the *Vedanta*.

That evening they had visiting the *ashram* a petite, soft-spoken lady, steeped in Vedantic truths, her life one of dedication and love. Vandana Mataji had a quaint little *ashram* in Rishikesh, having taught various nuns, naming the Himalayas as her source and resource. She kept me enthralled with her recounts of my favourite Vietnamese monk, Tich Nhat Hanh. She would mimic him affectionately, and I was falling over with laughter when I felt the presence of a man come and sit by me. Taming my laughter and questions a bit, throwing a glance his way, he caught my eye and whispered, "Shambhavi? I am Swami Veda Bharati."

Unable to recognise him, since he had shaved his beard, taking away several years from his appearance, I shot up and bowed to him in reverence. He smiled softly and we shared beautiful words of wisdom. A *swami*, whose faith had a much deeper insight had been illustrated beautifully in his profound writings. He invited me to spend time at his *ashram* to seek knowledge from the sacred texts.

My favourite place in my travels all over the world is the Glass House by the flowing River Ganga, where I meditated and healed, rejuvenating my soul. The surroundings were in tandem with the gentle vibrations of the Universe. The cottages are set among *lichee* and mango orchards that run alongside silvery sand beaches interspersed with boulders and rocks neceding into the aquamarine waters of the Ganga.

Uttara was my favourite cottage, where I enjoyed my showers in the open air, watching the Ganga flow under the preening rays of sunshine through the dark foliage above. During the night showers, my body would revel in the sweet *soma* of the moonlight that played truant against my wet skin. Sensuality surpassed every subtle nuance, bringing about an aura of ecstatic bliss. The nights lulled one into a deep sleep to the powerful rush of the waters.

As a surreal full Moon was shining through the wafting dark clouds,

The Silence of Ramana Maharshi

I made my way to the beach to perform a full night of *sadhana*, standing immersed in the flow of the Ganga. The glow of candles dug into the sand creating an illumined magic and holding me spellbound! The luminescence of the full Moon, its bright light reflected in the flowing waters, and the strong sound of the rush of the waves rendered me invisible to the landscape, merging me into its surreality.

Nikhil Arjun, my elder son, had decided to sit watchful by me on the beach, worrying that I would be carried away by the powerful currents in my hypnotic state of meditation. His caring created the ambience of lit candles for me. Sons can be wonderful, most times!

Eclipses cause strange forces and are excellent for *sadhana* as the gravitational effects multiply the effect of the *puja* being performed or *mantra japa* being chanted. If one does 100 repetitions of a *mantra* during an eclipse, it is like doing 1,00,000 *japas* on an ordinary day. Nothing compares to the power of this moment for offering prayers or oblations or rites for deceased ancestors.

In India, festivals occur with special forms of worship at these specific times. These energised times were specified by the *rishis* in order to help the *sadhakas* to gain deeper perceptions. One should not waste a single moment during an eclipse. *Sadhana* on the banks of a river or any large body of water, especially immersing one's body in the waters while meditating, is very auspicious at such moments.

However, these time-periods that create so much power and energy can also have negative effects on the human mind, so certain precautions must be taken. One should never look at an eclipse because the rays emitted from the eclipse have a disturbing effect on the mind. Moreover, a pregnant woman should remain indoors during the eclipse, lest the powerful rays affect her unborn child. Food or water should not be taken during the period of the eclipse, and preferably up to 12 hours before and after it.

Besides eclipses there are four extremely potent nights, ideal for performing *sadhana* and rituals. The first is Maha Shivaratri, the great night of Shiva, which falls every year on the night before the new moon during the lunar month of *Magha*, end February or early March. On

Shivaratri, people try to stay awake all night long. It is believed Shiva will come, just for a moment, to the one who does not fall asleep even for a moment. But Shiva is too adroit for us mortals, and almost everyone who stays up all night, nods off for at least a moment or so just when Shiva is nearest.

The second is Kruraratri, the cruel night, which is the festival of Holi, the next full Moon after Maharatri. As the cruel night comme-morates the burning to death of the demoness Holika, this night is conducive to the practitioners of black magic. Then follows Moharatri, the night of delusion or Krishna's birth-night before Janamashtmi, meant for the worship of Krishna, falling in the month of August. Krishna deluded everyone with His play of *maya*. The last is Kalaratri, the black night or the new Moon night just before Diwali.

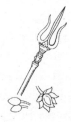

Maha Shivaratri, the Night of Bliss

'Om namo namaha Shiva shivaaya namo namaha.'

One Maha Shivaratri I stayed up all night paying obeisance to the *Shivalingam*. Worship of the *lingam* helps one connect with one's own divine being. Simultaneously Shiva in his personal form touches the soul of the worshipper gradually until we experience the divine truth, his *darshana*. I prepared myself for this special night with a deep excitement, putting together all the ingredients for the *puja*.

My sacred space was heavy with the aroma of intoxication, the leaves of the hemp, cannabis plant commonly called *bhang*, Shiva's holy plant, the triune leaf of the *bel*, *bilva* or wood-apple tree. This threefold leaf is the symbol of the triune God, the threefold nature of the Universe, the three *gunas* of *sattva*, *rajas* and *tamas*, the trinity of creation, sustenance and dissolution. There were also the white funnel-shaped flowers of the *dhatura*, thorn apple, symbolically sounding the trumpet of salvation, and their thorny fruits, three of which I placed at my altar as an offering to Shiva. The white lotus and the *kusa* grass were there as well, and personally I made the offering of red roses, expressing my passionate nature.

I bathed, preparing myself for the wonders of the night, oiling and perfuming my body, leaving my damp dark stresses to flow down my shoulders. My eyes deepened with the dark shadow of kohl, my lips stained with red, draping my naked body with the passion play of red Chanderi enhanced with gold *zari* woven intricately into its borders, tying it in the tribal-style sari leaving the shoulders bare.

The tinkle of my antique, *todar* silver *payals* fastened at my ankles, the waist chain with the *matsya*, fish, clinking at the sway of the waist, I made the *tilak* of *bhasma*, holy ash, on my forehead and the *tripunda*, the three horizontal lines at my throat, followed by the *sindoor*, red vermillion, at the centre of the forehead and the nape of my neck.

Mine is a simple worship that entails following only a few basic rules through the strains of my heart. Readying myself for performing the *homa*, I gently moved into the deep night, chanting my *mantras* to the ardent flames, finishing at half past three. Having placed the *havan kund* outside on the terrace for the embers to cool off, I heard the sound of thunder rolling and lightning flashing in the sky. Was this the play of Shiva-Shakti?

I always take these as signs from Shiva communicating with me. Rushing out to bring in the *havan kund*, I felt drops of rain on my face and arms, standing outside for a while receiving His blessings. Past four in the morning, I began to feel drowsy, so I lit some more incense and filled the lamp with *ghee*. By five I readied myself for sleep, unable to stay awake.

No signs of Shiva! I was surprised and disappointed, having reasoned with my heart that my Lord had so many more devoted *sadhakas* to visit that he would come to me another time. With His name on my lips and in my heart, I fell off to sleep. Waking up at eight in the morning, I lit some incense and smiled to myself. How would He have been able to pass me by?

Yes! Shiva had come and taken a piece out of the *dhatura* fruit, my offering to Him. Excitement gripped my heart. I was too nervous to

Maha Shivaratri, the Night of Bliss

pick it up, though later in the day I placed some of the seeds that had rolled out into my mouth as *prasada* and kept the rest away. I was in a state of *ksiva*, one who is intoxicated with Divinity.

Shiva brought out the little girl's quest for love, the deep love that I seemed to evade, my need to make conversation with Ma and ask Her my list of questions. I guess She was consciously avoiding this constant prattle. I enjoyed my solitude, wanting to stay away from other people so as to enable me to forget myself. I remained celibate through choice, conserving the *ojas*, the essence of physical energy, which enhances our aura and immunity. My beautiful men-friends remained close to me and the ones with baser values fell away. Life has a beautiful way of removing the chaff once you begin walking the path of divinity. One never really loses the zest for living; life is still wild and exuberant with a conscious reality.

Every step was a *sadhana*, offering whatever I did to Shiva. Faith became the key to open the gates to heaven, turning my entire existence over to the higher powers; this was the essence of my *sadhana*. Never having believed in renouncing everything, I still made my mistakes, committed follies, experienced heartbreak and disillusionment. But I never gave up, never! Spirituality sometimes has connotations of a child's play: sometimes I was childlike, other times, Ma played games with me. We must never lose the childlike fervour and zest in reaching the ultimate goal.

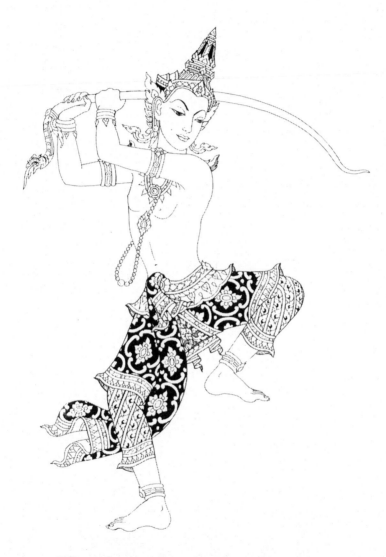

Timelessness of Life and Death
on the *Ghats* of Kashi

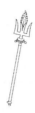

Life and Death are the Rhythms of Time

'Life and death are the rhythms of time, the ebb and flow of the eternal sea. Kali is the life that exists in death and the death that exists in life...'

The Indian city of Varanasi or Kashi is a spiritual amalgamation of ancient, medieval and modern India. It is a seeker's treasure-cove of both the left-hand and right-hand *Tantra*. Every seeker here receives illumination, a dousing of mysticism, and perception of the Ultimate Reality. The city pulsates with both life and death; nowhere else in the world will this be experienced simultaneously. Yet Kashi cannot be written about merely as history, it's about timelessness, not just unfolding the cycle of birth and death. The city pulsates with the longings, prayers, breath and sweat of millions of people and visitors from all over the world.

The crowded, narrow streets echo the cries of death and the music of the divinity of humanity experiencing the struggles and temptations in the mesh of *maya*, illusion. Smoke filled with the essence of sandalwood, *samagri* kneaded into *ghee* and the singe of burnt flesh wafting through the warm breeze, rising above the waters of the Ganga create a universal mystique that has to be experienced and is indescribable. Generations of the devout come here to offer libations to the departed, offering *pindas* or balls of rice to propitiate the *pitris,* the ancestral spirits.

During the evening I'd take a boat and move down the river watching the evening *arati,* the ritual offering. In a row, young priests in crisp white *dhotis,* bare bodied would perform the ceremony illuminating the night sky with the camphor-lit fire, flashing plumes through the air to the chant of powerful Vedic *mantras.* The illumination of the reflected fires lit up the Ganga waters, finding expression in celestial calligraphic formations. It was captured vividly through my camera in photographs. The deities seemed to be speaking to me through these currents, conveying their grace.

Death took on a mystical·reality for me very early in life, and this reality was experienced on the *ghats* of Kashi. The *ghats* are alive all through the day and night, with no silent respite from either the vendors calling, or Vedic chants, devotional renderings, the strains of music from the courtesans' gaudy interiors or the sharp crackle of fiery flames emanating from pyres. Yes, even the courtesan dances her role sensuously for the ardent lovers, relentlessly giving the message of the ephemeral nature of pleasure and the futility of attachment. Every aspect of life and death transcends its potentiality.

My fear of death took a lot of introspection before I learnt to deal with its ponderous meaning. I spent hours sitting at the *ghats* watching human bodies being confined to the fire. Even here, in one's final moments, man cheated upon his brethren, literally dragging his half-burnt corpse and flushing it down the flow of the Ganga, greedy to take over the next pyre. Our last rites are not even spared from such callousness.

Varanasi is the city of Shiva, the Cosmic Lord, manifesting as the destroyer, but in the role of *Ishvara,* He grants us grace and protection for He is Creator and sustainer as well. As destroyer, He doesn't destroy the soul, but only the world of His illusion. Everything that is bound by time must perish, and by freeing man from time, Shiva renders us timeless.

Death is most unexpected, unless one is evolved enough to envision its nearness, and there is no way to bargain with it! Our mind is of the view that birth is the coming into being of that which did not previously exist and death is its ending. Looking deeply at its perspective, we clearly see that our understanding about birth and death is untrue.

No phenomenon whatsoever can come into existence out of nothing. Every action is ceaselessly transforming itself in due course of time that it traverses. The cloud doesn't die away; it merely turns into rain. The rain is not born; it is only the transformation and continuation of the cloud. Nature in its forms of flowers and fruits, human emotions of joy and sorrow — all conform to this principle of no-birth and no-death. To believe that after death we no longer exist is a very narrow view.

Life is suffering, but it is also wonderful! Death, heartbreak, pain and sorrow are unavoidable in our life's experience. But if our understanding is deep and our mind set free, we can learn to accept these realities with tranquillity, and the ensuing suffering will be greatly lessened. This is not to say that we should close our eyes and not experience this suffering, but by merely remaining in contact with the suffering and not fighting it, we give rise to and nourish our own natural love and compassion. Suffering becomes the element that nourishes our deep love and compassion, and we learn to face it unafraid.

Sometimes we stop appreciating the small miracles of everyday life — a glass of clear water quenching the thirst, a rainbow highlighting the hues of a spectrum of colours, the golden sunset, the cool breeze playing with our hair, a step taken in freedom! We have so much to be happy for, yet we grow up looking at life with disdain. The Universe mirrors our inner image. If I look into the mirror searching for fine lines of age, they'll be there, but if I see the soft glow of maturity as a reflection of my years, it gets enhanced making me beautiful beyond my years.

Nowhere in the world does one's illusory existence stare you in the face as in Kashi — the lure of the vendor's cries of temptation, to the array of intricately woven designs into rich silk dyed to brilliant hues of the rainbow, the display and tinkle of delicate glass bangles, rays of the sun caught off tangent gleaming from the surface of brass and copper pots, the gold and brass spires of the temples highlighting the skyline and the aroma of sweet-smelling coconut water flowing from half broken coconut offerings. It is here, in Varanasi, that the Ganga turns its direction in its flow for a short distance northwards, towards her origin, curving like a crescent Moon, like the diadem sparkling in Shiva's dreadlocks.

I was still very much a part of this *maya*, working with the weavers, designing brocades for a holiday collection for my favourite men's wear designer, Joseph Abboud, into whose fold I was introduced when he ventured to launch his home-ware collection. The man responsible for some of my most soulful work was the tall, handsome, sensitive Victor Hollingsworth. I arrived in New York with my first collection of home textiles, in which I had played subtly with masculine textures of herringbone stitch, Houndstooth weaves in shades of steel grey and Earth, sensuously juxtaposed with pewter silk tissue. Passion flowed into the rich burgundy weaves of paisley to decorate a wedding table of a fashionable catalogue.

We just seemed to understand each other and I loved creating collections with him. Victor seemed to exist with a childlike raciness. He'd excitedly walk me down to the stores on Fifth Avenue to show me my designs exhibited in show-windows, beds laid out with the intermingling of textures, subtle natural linen, combined with the purity of pintucked white organdie sheathed with silver silk tissue. This too was intoxicating — the euphoria of power, success, desire, and beauty. To evolve one must experience the grind of every aspect of life, to understand what *maya*, illusion, is all about, only then can we make our choices. This is where I learned to experience life with passion, a passion that would find its other-worldly flowering in Kashi.

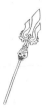

My Experience with a *Tantric*

'Shakti roop ko maram na payo, shakti gayi tab man pachhitayo.'
– Durga Chalisa :32
(Since he did not realise your immense glory, his powers waned and
thence he repented.)

Experiences enrich our lives and open secret doors to the unknown, mysterious ways of life. I was working closely with Karunesh, spending a lot of time traversing the narrow streets, in and out of weaver's homes, designing my textiles. He had a great sense of humour and was a bit of a rebel, sporting long, black, wavy hair. He decided to introduce me to a *Tantric* whom he visited regularly. I was curious to experience the powers of a *Tantric* to know what their mystique was all about. We arrived at this house, rather dimly lit late in the evening and found myself facing a tall, slim man with large, intense eyes, probably in his sixties.

He connected with me and we got drawn into a conversation about the dark goddess, when he suddenly asked me to come and sit right in front of him. A shiver went through my spine; there was something deep and dark about the atmosphere; the red naked bulb above a picture of Ma Kali was exuding redness into the dimness of the room. The mistrusting mind always becomes cautious, and I had instructed my escort at no point to ever leave me alone with the *Tantric*, literally threatening him into submission.

I was unusually dressed in a Shiva T-shirt with an over shirt and a sarong. The T-shirt had a story to tell as well. Driving through Santa Fe, we stopped outside a quaint shopping place and I wound my way through the shops into a boutique. It was most unlike me, for I rarely shop for clothes. The corner seemed to draw me in, and there was hanging this solitary T-shirt with Shiva beautifully painted on it. His half open eyes spoke volumes to me, his face expressing a serene gentleness behind the immense power of the Universe. Shiva seemed to save my day. The *Tantric* bent low and asked me to remove my over shirt. My legs began to tremble, fear seeming to take over me entirely, realising that I had made a mistake by trying to.be too adventurous.

Removing the shirt, I shut my eyes, brought all my attention to my third eye, and began chanting my *guru mantra*. The intensity of concentration was so strong that I held on to my own, not succumbing to his *Tantric mantras*. An eerie numbness set in and a strong sense of power came over me; my body drew calm, the trembling had stopped. The *Tantric* was getting agitated and announced to my escort what a powerful lady I was. Something snapped in me and opening my eyes to see him in a trance-like state, I stood up, mumbled something and decided to leave.

My escort was now trembling with nervousness and was slow to start the two-wheeler scooter. He was silent and kept apologising. Reaching the safe confines of my room, I went in for a hot shower and sat in meditation, actually able to visualise the *Tantric* pacing up and down his room in a fiery stupor. The next morning, he contacted me in the hotel, asking me to drop by and visit him on my way to the airport. I didn't want to appear disrespectful and did drop by to be told by his son how his father had consumed alcohol and was pacing the house the entire night trying to create a *tabeez*, a locket for me. He placed it round my neck and I headed for the airport to catch my flight home, very nearly playing with my life.

Within a matter of two-and-a-half hours, I began to go slightly numb. By the time I reached home, all life seemed to be draining out of me. Silently I lay down and began to drift away, when I heard the phone ring faintly by my bedside. I spoke into it and was telling Hari in New York of my experience with the *Tantric* and that I was beginning to feel like I was dying. In his panic, he asked me if I was wearing anything given by the *Tantric*. In a distantly faint voice, I heard him instruct me to take the *tabeez* off my neck. I never seemed to know how I managed to pull it off my neck, but the phone slipped away from my hand drifting me into listless blackness.

It was late evening when my mother came in to awaken me. I had grown a paler shade of white. There was no explanation to render to the look of panic in her eyes. Getting myself together, drawing courage from my prayers, I managed to sit up. The next morning I took the *tabeez* and immersed it in River Yamuna, watching the waves absorb its magic. I had learnt my lesson. Ever since, I stay away from the magic of *Tantrics*.

The Grandmotherly Spirit

'Perceived as the void, as the dissolved form of consciousness, when all beings are dissolved in sleep in the supreme Brahman, having swallowed the entire Universe, the seer-poets call her the most glorious, Dhumavati.'
– Ganapati Muni, Uma Sahasram

Dhuma, literally translates as 'smoke', but smoke, like fire, has many mystic meanings. Ma Dhumavati came into my existence obscuring all else, throwing me off guard, sending me reeling with the impact of Her appearance. It was during September, four days before the autumnal Navaratri when I was performing my weekly ritual of the Monday visit to the Navagraha temple near Sarojini Market. A temple built in the traditional south Indian style, the central deity was Vinayaka, Lord Ganapati.

The young boy selling flowers had grown accustomed to my face and would joyously fill my arms with flowers for offering, with some to take home. If I ever missed a Monday *darshan*, he would cheekily query my whereabouts. The priests hailed from the south, with shy demeanour and smiling eyes. My eyes rested on a particular *pujari*, seemingly lost in the venerations to the Lord. He was youthful, and stately, the *vibhuti* markings of Lord Shiva lending awe to his bare torso.

Over a year of familiarity, and with curiosity finally taking him over, he approached me shyly, asking, "Are you an *aghori*?"

I smiled at him, replying, "Don't each of us, in the passion of Shiva, have a streak of the *aghori*?"

His eyes would light up whenever he saw me, the sparkle of a zillion twinkles from the illumination of the fire *arati*. Who knows when and where there was a connection with some gentle resonance prevailing!

My ritual was to pay obeisance to Lord Ganapati, offer him a garland rich with red, red roses, moist with the sprinkle of water and a coconut. The time was of *sandhya*, dusk, ushering in the darkness of night. The *arati* was the highlight amidst the powerful chanting and fire offering.

I would pay obeisance to the *navagrahas*, with deep admiration for the lords of the nine planets, dressed in the colour of their nature, decorated with flowers. Strangely though, I would skip the altar of Anjaneya, not having had a rapport with his mysticism up to that point.

One Monday, I was guided to his altar to bow before him. Standing in silence, gentleness and great strength seemed to be emanating through him. He was dressed in the exuberance of orange silk, a garland with a hundred, bright green, betel leaves draped around his being and red roses strewn at his feet.

A flow of sensations seemed to enter through my feet, numbing my being into a revered silence, shutting my eyes to the world around me. With folded hands placed before my *anahata chakra*, the heart reached out in silent blessings, when before me appeared the form of an elderly woman, draped with a white cloth covering her head. Her face was deeply etched with lines of times gone by, hair dishevelled. She never seemed to cause any fears of alarm, though the deep charcoal glow in her eyes seemed to pierce through my heart. There was a gentleness and warmth exuding through her.

I desperately wanted to see beyond this obscurity, this visionary old myth. I opened my eyes and Lord Anjaneya warmly embraced my soul. My palms must have opened to receive His grace, for I came into my being sensing a cold flow of water into them. Awakened from my stupor of experience, I gently accepted the flow of the holy water offering being poured into my hands by the *pujari*, the temple priest.

Shiva was awaiting my obeisance to Him, so I walked away to the shelter of the widespread *pipal*, banyan tree, sheltering the *Shivalingam* enthroned with flowers and his favourite *bilva* leaves, steadily moistened and cooled by the overhead flow of water. He always calmed my being with His powerful grace; my hands would quiver to His touch, with a silent prayer on my lips. 'Show me the way, O Lord!'

The last stop was at the feet of Naganath, standing in the brilliance of his five-hooded spread, the coils running smoothly to Mother Earth. Sometimes the serpent Lord would glimmer from the glow of the small, lit earthen lamps reflecting the mustard oil offering. I prayed in silence to Vasuki, the Serpent-god. Once a year I would offer the sweet milk of the tender coconut, pouring it gently over the splendour of *Naga Devata*.

Dhumavati, representing the grandmotherly spirit, is the great teacher who bestows the ultimate lessons of birth and death on her *sadhakas*. Her nature through the mirage of smoke is not of illumination, but one of obscuration. Yet by obscuring all that is known, she reveals another — the depth of the unknown.

Dhumavati represents the negative powers of life: disappointment, frustration, humiliation, defeat, loss and sorrow, the experiences which overpower the ordinary mind. To the yogi these experiences open the doors of opportunity to realise the reality, which transcends all desire.

She represents the darkness of primordial ignorance. Yet ignorance has a higher meaning, for only when we accept that we are ignorant that we will truly begin to learn, which enables us to forget or let go of all fears, desires, opinions and beliefs. She is also the primal smoke out of which all creation arises, the galactic cloud from which the stars emerge. Her smoke is both the way in and out of all the mysteries of light and darkness.

As Vamadeva Shastri has described her as one among the *Dasha Mahavidya* goddesses and as one with "the glowing face of a wise matriarch, knowing all the trials and tribulations of life. On a cosmic level, she is the primordial smoke, the cloud of unknowing from which the Universe arises and into which it eventually returns. She grants the power to unfocus our consciousness from its attachment to the details of the outer world, to its greater focus on the infinite expanse of consciousness. In that all the solidity of the external world dissolves into a haze of smoke, a cloud in the sky of the mind. From her standpoint, life is just a dance of clouds in the void. She is the reflection of the elder form of *agni* or fire, which is also the inextinguishable flame of pure being, out of which the Universe rises like smoke. Yet it is a smoke of incense with a fragrance that permeates all the time and opens all the *nadis* of the heart."

That night, I devoured all the precious information on Ma Dhumavati in Vamadeva's poetic expression from the depths of a heart familiar with the goddess's love, bringing my night to a close with her powerful *mantra* obscuring the false lights and creating a protective smoke around us.

'Dhum dhum Dhumavati svaha!'

Cosmic Fires Smear Me with Ash

'Yet the timeless in you is aware of life's timelessness,
and knows that yesterday is but today's memory and
tomorrow is today's dream.'
– Kahlil Gibran

Shiva manifests as *vibhuti bhushan*, He who is bedecked with ash-marks. He wanders in cremation grounds amidst blazing pyres and, smearing His body with *bhasma*, ash, is known as *Bhasmeshvar*, the Lord of ash. To the celestial ascetic, every joy, every sorrow, each birth and death will eventually end up in its own funeral pyre. After every fire, only ash will remain, so where is the need for all this pain, anger and greed? One must exist in eternal *vairagya*, timeless equanimity.

Vibhuti in Sanskrit translates into wealth, bestowing the ash-smeared *sadhaka* with all kinds of abundance. The applying of *vibhuti* induces in us the thought of ashes as the end of the body and the ephemeral condition of everything in this world with the exception of the Lord. *Vibhuti* is held as most sacred and connects us to our essence.

Bhasma is the holy ash prepared from the *homa*, a sacrificial fire, with special wood from the *pipal* and *khair* (catechu) trees along with *ghee*, honey, incense and herbs. It is a special offering for the worship of the Lord. The word *bhasma* indicates "that by which our sins are destroyed and remembering the Lord". My morning ritual involves applying *vibhuti* and then *sindoor*, the red vermillion, as a gesture of obeisance and protection.

Some day I contemplated connecting with a man who has tended to and played with the cosmic fire himself, understanding its role in the whirlpool of existence. Not necessarily the fire itself! There still is a lot of smouldering in the coals that has to settle down.

My Mevlana has said, "*Agni* is the guru and the master within. All the *agnis* have their place and must be understood. The greatest of the *rishis*, the *Angirasas* or sons of *agni* (Brihaspati or Jupiter is the foremost of these) are born of his coals. One must become *agni* to truly teach, yet also to really learn. From the union of Shiva and Shakti comes *agni*. Yet *agni* also brings about the union of Shiva and Shakti."

The *Durga sukta* (Vedic hymn to Durga) begins, "For *agni* we press out the *soma*" (*jatavedase sunavama soma*). Durga is born of *agni*. She arises from the *soma* offered to Shiva, which also creates its own sacred ash.

Fire is an awesome force to reckon within us, capable of creating a higher passion as well as burning up our lower passions — a process symbolised by the sacred ash. Gradually fire drew me into its fold. I began to study its nature and to use it in performing *homa*, the sacred fire ceremony in Vedic rites. Blazing fire is a powerful element. Through visualisation, we can request the outer flames to enter within us and enkindle the inner fire of the subtle body, which when ignited helps us progress through our *sadhana*. The fire of the *homa* will gradually burn away all our limitations in the body and mind, consuming our negative *karmas*.

Interestingly, I approached the fire through the heart, developing my own ceremony, wanting it to unfold its own passion within me. I wrote down the steps of how I wanted to perform the *homa*, taking guidance from Vedic ritual books. I had the procedure translated into Sanskrit through a scholarly principal of a school in the remote Himalayan abode of Kanatal — Shastriji — as we addressed him.

My first experience with the *homa* was filled with mirth, yet with all earnestness as well. It was performed on a full Moon night in the open farmlands belonging to a friend. A clearing was sought out, the Earth damp from previous watering.

The overhead Moon seemed to beckon us to begin. We tried to get all the steps performed correctly, reading in torchlight. Meanwhile, my friend was translating it into Hindi for the benefit of the two Bahadurs, the Nepalese helping hands, who wanted to understand what we were doing. The *havan* came to a close with an offering of coconuts, symbolising the subconscious mind, to the *agni*, the fire. Three coconuts and our three subconscious minds seem to crowd the mid-sized *havan kund* (fire-altar), bursting forth their sweet milk into the flames of the fire. My moment of silent happiness was acknowledged by a beautiful owl, which flew in as a witness for the goddess.

Those were days of sheer confusion among a particular circle of acquaintances. Much drama was played out, human emotions weaving a fabric through a warp and weft of unethical, improper displays of passions bordering on a game of roulette. The finer nuances of love and truth were rendered into the starry nights through the lilting songs of my friend Nasir. Life is a multi-dimensional journey — some moving on and others remaining static, happy in their world of *maya*, taking their turns on the merry-go-rounds of life.

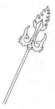

Tapas, the Fire of Spiritual Aspiration

'Prayatnah sadhakah.'
- Siva Sutra 2.2
(A seeker is one who makes an effort.)

Tapas is an intense yogic practice. It is often simply translated as asceticism and can be confused with bizarre practices like standing on one leg for long periods of time, or taking to long fasts.

Yet, real *tapas* is more than any enforced asceticism. It is the heat that arises from a passionate form of the Divine energy seeking to transcend all limitations. *Tapas* is the heat of spiritual inquiry and aspiration that makes the *sadhaka* consume all the fleeting needs and desires in life. The fire in the soul connects with the life-fire in the body, finding expression through the heart, leading one to liberate or detach oneself from illusion, creating the way to self-realisation. This is the real inner movement of *tapas*.

David Frawley throws light on *tapas* as the form of Bhairavi, the warrior-goddess, representing Divine anger and wrath. She is the supreme power of speech, which has the nature of fire. This means that the goddess herself is the real energy of *tapas*, which is her power of purification and transformation. True *tapas* is guided by the goddess.

It is part of Uma's offering to Shiva. It is not just a matter of doing something difficult for its own sake.

Illusion or *maya* can produce many obstacles, sometimes creating a subtle 'ego'. On the spiritual path, many so-called gurus or *sadhakas* create certain boundaries describing the path in fixed terms or outer behavioural patterns and look to these outer appearances as the main thing. Typical examples of this are abstinence from meat, sex or even alcohol and smoking, as if such outer marks of renunciation were enough to indicate the existence of the inner fire.

Abstinence may be beneficial — to be free from smoking and eating meat can be conducive to one's spiritual growth. However, such outer changes have little value if there is no real fire burning within. If a person applies such outer forms as an end in themselves, it can bring about a fanaticism or even arrogance, trying to portray oneself as above or different from others. I don't think someone eating meat or drinking alcohol or making love is necessarily 'unholy'.

Even vegetarians or non-smokers can be brutal in their behaviour in relationship to mankind, expressing 'unholy' traits in how they see others in their hearts. People cannot be judged according to these relative habits. There are no simple outer criteria for assessing the degree of someone's enlightenment. Most important is to see to what extent a person lives in true love, experiencing harmony with the higher consciousness. This is also a kind of *tapas*.

The *aghori* overcomes every human limitation by dealing with every human restraint, every aspect of human life, which allows one to exist at the expense of other beings. We can appreciate the light of altruism only when we have experienced the darkness of selfishness and negativity. The *aghori* takes every possible experience and turns it into devotion of the great Mother Goddess. The *tapas* of an *aghori* is a *tapas* without boundaries, but which can burn up all limitations.

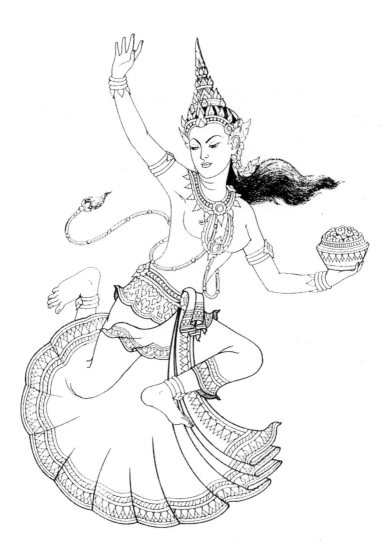

Angels, *Devas* and
Higher Frequencies

The Wisdom of Knowing the Difference

'Grant me the serenity to accept the things I cannot change,
the courage to change the things I can,
and the wisdom to know the difference.'

Spiritual experiences are very personal, private occurrences that happen in everyone's lives. Angels are not mythical beings or projections of the unconscious mind. Angels are real; they have their own personalities and characteristics. Angels are a source of empowerment that help us connect with our higher self, the soul.

A spiritual awakening unlike anything experienced earlier seemed to overcome me during the turn of the millennium. Many realised souls shared a similar experience with me. I personally experienced these vibrations in deep meditation on the banks of River Chenab, having retreated to this solitary beautiful place with my family and friends, with the single thought of meditating under the last setting Sun of the millennium through the night, remaining awake to view the first rays of the rising Sun of the year 2000, with spurts in between, fervently trying to capture the time on camera.

As the profuse rays of the last setting Sun threw eclectic golden reflections in the fast-flowing tide of the river, I surrendered myself to the confines of the magical Universe, experiencing an abundance of blessings from the higher powers. I was consciously aware of the prevailing vibrations around me, my being rendering the chants of the *Gayatri mantra* right through the transition of the millennium, the moments ticking between the two phases of the Sun.

The deep pink glow of the first rising Sun of the new millennium shone upon us, gradually filling its space on the far horizon. I thought to myself, 'I have a beautiful journey ahead. This is only the beginning!' Throughout the chanting of the *Gayatri mantra*, a continuous silent process began to stir deep within me. Along with the combined forces of the blessings of Ma Gayatri, the potent vibrations prevailing in the Universe of the time passing on from one to the next millennium, my life too was coming a full circle.

And as time passed me by through the coming year, it was November and Thanksgiving, and having stayed back for an unknown reason in New York, another breathtaking time was experienced. We'd stroll down the avenues, taking in the myriad twinkling lights, the windows tempting us lesser mortals with Christmas delights, the cold winds playing across our faces. It was fairytale like. Engulfed by the raptures of success, beauty and creativity I had gained that year, I was abundantly joyous.

Over a trussed up turkey and a lot of laughter and warmth, I grew aware of a tall gentleman watching me. After dinner, my hostess Kathy wanted guidance with my pendulum, which I had learned to use to bring in messages from higher powers. We retreated to the corridor and sat on the floor. Kathy began asking all her questions and I sought guidance from my pendulum for answers. I began delving into the unknown.

The tall presence came and sat down beside me on the floor. "Hi! I'm Joseph Dumas. I have a message for you. It is from your grandmother." I looked at him perplexed and he continued nonetheless with the message, completely lost into another space and time. He was in a trance, and I seemed to be getting goosebumps. He clearly described my maternal grandmother, told me about how and when she died, which was at a very young age.

Nana, as we lovingly called her, was of Scottish descent and a truly blessed soul. I remember my mother narrating an incident when she was young, how Nana, in the streets of Chinatown in Kolkata, had stopped a tonga-puller, the driver of a buggy drawn by a horse, dragged the man to the floor and taking the whip from his hand, use it on him. The man was stunned for he was merrily whipping his poor horse. It was a sight watching this four-foot nothing woman with flaming red hair use the whip. She always had sympathy for the underdog.

Joseph continued to narrate incidents from my own marriage of deep anguish and times that were to come. He clearly explained a paradigm shift would come about in my life and a deep spiritual connection would be made. I would take to healing ways, and would have a large following — though all this seemed other worldly to me at the moment.

My friends Hari and Kathryn were taken aback and fell completely silent. They all knew me as a happy girl, filled with a zest for life. I too, was quite shaken by the whole experience, for here was a complete stranger conveying my life through the medium of my grandmother! The most beautiful part was that Nana was my guardian angel and always by my side. We drove home in silence. Hari busied himself with making some coffee on reaching home. Sitting down, he placed a hand around my shoulders and we both cried silently, living out our own deep painful sorrows, allowing them to heal through our outbursts of tears.

And I began communing with Nana and the other angels. Angels are real; my own experience tells me so. During the heart-breaking experience of September eleventh at the Twin Towers, Joseph reached out to me once again. He had two friends caught in the burning inferno. He described the women and asked me to meditate and help rescue them as they were dying, frightened souls. Sitting in deep meditation, I saw they had moved on to another dimension, and I prayed deeply for their souls to be freed from all fear, for I could feel their terror and couldn't sleep for days.

Needing to heal myself, as there were still the insecurities and pain of a marriage run into turbulent times, of love having gone awry, of

151

confusion and deep despair, I sought the angels' healing guidance in order to shift my vibrational frequency to its highest and subtlest rate. The angels guide us to make this shift as a process of 'ascension'. When we truly realise and experience the knowledge of discovering oneness with God or our higher self, we are in the state of ascension. Angels want us to increase our frequency so as to be better suited to the upcoming shift of spiritual vibrations on the planet, and to adapt to a changing world by giving us energy and guidance.

The higher our frequency, the more we will be intuitively aware of pending earthly changes, in the way the animal kingdom can foresee earthquakes and natural calamities. Our high-frequency bodies will be able to withstand events that would traumatise denser, lower frequency bodies.

The angels help us through signs and signals, Divine guidance, and by intervening in our lives. They help us maintain a peaceful mind. The angels can guide us heal our relationship problems, if we ask for their help. Yogic thought also recognises such angels as special groups of guiding *devas* and *gandharvas*. They are among the subtle companions of the human race; they are our inner friends that we need to access once more if we want to truly progress as a species.

Prayers, Love and Light

'And if it is for your comfort to pour your darkness into space,
it is also for your delight to pour forth the dawning of your heart.'
- Kahlil Gibran

Prayer is a very powerful way to connect with the heavenly forces for the purpose of healing. Love is already existent and pervasive deep within us. We surely don't need another person in our lives in order to feel loved. But the expression of true love expressed from one person to another brings about a deep satisfaction for the soul. Angels are interested in helping us reach and sustain happy soul relationships at all levels.

A wonderful prayer of healing for each of us to hold in our hearts is the simple calling, 'Thy will be done.' With these words we can rest assured that the supreme power is taking care of everything and we can save ourselves from endless worry.

Archangel Raphael has the green healing light, which heals all aspects of our physical challenges as pain, anguish and suffering. He releases all fear and darkness from within our beings.

Projecting a 'white light' is a magical way to ensure the safety and stability of our beings and our surroundings. The white light is an angel of energy that has life-force or *pranic* energy and an intelligence of its own, which creates a shield that ensures us protection. Simply close your eyes and visualise a 'white light' surrounding the entire outline of the person or object. Once one is able to visualise this eggshell of white light completely covering oneself in the mind's eye, the task is complete and we are safe within its field of protection.

New Delhi can be magical at times, amidst the chaos of traffic and noise. The grandeur of historical monuments, carrying the vibrations of civilisations of bygone years, paved the way for my mystical moments. In the heart of the city, on a rooftop overlooking the golf course, was a quaint, sparsely furnished flat belonging to a friend. I affectionately referred to him as 'Daddo' and he called me Teerri, abbreviated from Titeeri, the name of a bird in northern India famous for its chatter and slim legs!

We'd spend many an evening watching the Sun set against the backdrop of the famed 'Qutab Minar' in the distance and the sensuous preening of masquerading peacocks on his rooftop. During the rains we'd watch them in their plumage-splendour to the musical strains of Nasir, who rendered old movie songs and *ghazals*. Those were wonderful moments. We'd sit into the wee small hours of the morning listening to him sing, watching the celestial play of the stars above.

It was in the early hours of dawn when before me appeared this beautiful angel, flying to and fro horizontally, in all her white diaphanous glory, and then appeared a huge mountain shape of white light with a shimmering outline gleaming in the dark night. Spellbound by the surreal wonder of this mythical apparition unfolding before me, the angel seemed to remain around me.

The only other time this angel appeared to me was in the cave of Adi Shankara, in Joshimath in the Himalayas, where I had stopped to stay a while in meditation. The cave was under the vast spread of a mulberry tree, with ancient carved statues of Nandi, Shiva's bull. The vibrations were alive, for while I closed my eyes to fall into a meditative state and before me floated this ethereal form of an angel in white, holding a torch ablaze, horizontally traversing the cave. The priest placed a beautiful marigold flower in the palms of my hands, which I carried with me to Delhi. It remained in its state of brilliance for over three weeks, without any water.

A woman with a child in her womb is always a deeply gratifying sight, the magical wonder of the phenomenon called womanhood. Sitting by my side on a flight to San Francisco was a woman with child. I am usually silent during my travels, using the time and space for inner work to be unfolded. We sat silently through the flight, when towards the end she turned to me and took my hand and placed a miniature version of the New Testament. "I want you to have this; it has been with me since I was a child." Her warm gesture touched me deeply. And both our eyes seemed to moisten, probably connecting to another shared lifetime.

Looking into the warmth of her eyes, I experienced a deep stirring within me, almost bringing a rush of tears brimming to my eyes. There seemed to be no words to explain my emotion, only feelings. We continued to sit by each other, sharing the calmness of silence. She must have been an earthly angel.

The angels usually try communicating with us by drawing our attention, sometimes using numbers, arranging meaningful sequences, drawing our attention to them. Most times a particular series will continuously be flashed either on a billboard, a clock, and a telephone number.

The numerical number, 111 in any arrangement, 1:11, 111 or 11 is telling us, "to monitor our thoughts carefully, being certain to only think what you want, not what you don't want. It is a sign that there is a gate opening up for opportunities and your thoughts are manifesting into form at a great speed. 111 is like a flashbulb, for the Universe has just taken a snapshot of your thoughts and is manifesting them into form."

It is a reminder that you are one with the Super Consciousness, God, and to experience the presence of the Creator's love within you. It also signifies that a situation has come a full circle.

Compassionate Messiah

'Even as the Son of Man came not to be served, but to serve,
and to give his life as a ransom for many. '
- Matthew 20:28

Kasauli is a quaint British cantonment at 6,000 ft in the Himalayan range of the Shimla hills, overlooking the stretch of broad avenues and boulevards laid down by Le Corbusier at Chandigarh in the plains. A magical panorama unfolds at night to the lights forming a mass of twinkling glowworms. These panoramic views must have caught the imagination of the late film director, Sir David Lean, the maker of classics like, '*The Bridge over the River Kwai*', '*Lawrence of Arabia*,' and '*Dr Zhivago*'. During the shooting of his film, '*A Passage to India*', in Kasauli he met the lovely Sandra Hotz, who lived there with her English parents and the two were married soon after.

In the summer months, my parents would come up with a brood of 16 greyhounds. It made a pleasurable sight watching these beautiful animals being taken for their walks off the beaten tracks. One summer, June Blossom miscarried her litter of pups and was feeling sad. We had the erstwhile authoress Ruth Jhabavala and her two daughters visit us every day to console the grieving mother. We enjoyed the blessings of a privileged childhood.

Growing up among a Christian Order of Nuns in a convent in a remote place in the Himalayas, we were very much influenced by them, and at the tender age of 13, I was inspired to become a nun — though, mind you I would have been a rather mischievous one, and probably broken every rule in the book! I grew very close to the Sisters, as we addressed them. One of them was lost in her inner world and I would always tell her, "You don't belong here; your eyes have the haze of another world." Soon she was called to the Vatican and we lost all contact with her.

As a young girl I would spend all my free time in the evenings, sitting on a hilltop at the back of our dining hall where the gardener nurtured his vegetables. Evenings I watched the Sun go down; its ardent play of rays ushered me into another world, becoming completely lost to my surroundings and at times not hearing the bell announcing a shift in the schedule. The nuns would worry about me and some would come and sit by me and open up their hearts. I was never lonely; alone yes, but I was happy and peaceful in being alone.

There were moments when I would feel myself floating above the Earth, flying in the skies, and would reason with myself, 'Could it simply be my hallucinations?' I still haven't fathomed the truth about my floating in air! I still believe I really did.

Jesus for me was never a vision seen only on the cross; He was always a compassionate, beautiful Messiah alive and moving amongst the people, healing, comforting, and caring with His gentle words, "Come unto me", speaks volumes from the heart, showing Him as a most magnanimously compassionate being, willing to take on the whole world's suffering into His heart. Love seemed to flow from His being.

The most touching narration for me was when Jesus visited the home of a woman, who in the eyes of the world was called a prostitute. When she poured precious perfume over His feet, Judas asked Jesus to stop her because much money was being wasted which could be given to help the poor. But Jesus said, "When I am gone there will always be poor people. You don't understand her heart. Let her do whatever she is doing." Jesus showed that Divine love does not exclude human love.

When invoking Him, I always seek an abundance of compassion. The most soulful picture of Jesus, with a piercing, heart-rending compassion flowing through His gaze, rests at my altar. He has the most beautiful eyes, brimming with sweetness and a gentle passion. I can never bring myself to stare into His eyes — they drive me crazy, just as the eyes of Maha Avatar Babaji and Ramana Maharshi do! There is an astounding presence of fervour in their depths.

I was deciding how to move around the pictures in my sacred space and felt Jesus might not be too happy with the company of Shiva, Ma Kali, and Maha Lakshmi. Lifting His picture to place it elsewhere, it began to reverberate in my hands. The vibrations were so powerful that I had to immediately place the picture back for fear of dropping it! What a co-existence — the deities, Messiahs and *siddhas* were perfectly happy sharing the same space. It is we lesser mortals who feel discomfort from the misconceptions created by our own inner minds, causing divisions and segregations not only between ourselves, but throughout this world. Some say Jesus was a yogi and came to India. Perhaps, he was. His energy seems comfortable among the Himalayas and *devatas* that dwell there.

In the year 2004, in the heat of a June morning, I lay myself on the bed, experiencing a fiery burning rising through the soles of my feet. I ran the Vipassana, meditation, through my being, trying to bring some calm through the feet into my body, when through a white light in my *ajna chakra*, the point between the eyebrows in the centre of the forehead, Jesus appeared to me — a beautiful vision of tenderness. His eyes penetrating my heart had tinges of a passionate pain and fervent compassion, seemingly filled with eternal truth and love. There was a white glow of light surrounding Him. What benign divinity! He was more splendrous than all the worldly pictures depicting Him. I feel He is despairingly trying to reach out to all of us to save His dream of a happy, loving, peaceful world, though I never perceived any hidden pain in His aura.

Sacrificing My Fire to the Ocean

'In the depths of your hopes and desires lies your silent
knowledge of the beyond.'
— Kahlil Gibran

Goa has golden moments for everyone I suppose, steeped as it is in history. The continuous process of waves brings in the even tide against the powerful backdrop of *Surya*, the Sun's omnipresence stirring up a certain zeal in our spirits. The fields running the length on either side of the road were a lush green, lined with tall coconut palms laden with fruit. We were a group of friends cruising along on the old Royal Enfield motorbikes, up to all the antics — standing up with hands thrown skywards in childlike exuberance. I can sum up the experience in one word — beatitude.

The powerful *yang* energy of the wide expanse of the ocean seemed to draw my *yin* energy into its grip, preparing me for the sacrifice of my inner fire into the waves of its oceanic fire. I threw all caution to Vayu, the Wind-god, truly making a ritual of offering the nudity of my body to its magnetic waves. I rode the waves, washing my soul, allowing them to take me into their fold, eventually floating in the stillness of the deep sea.

Awakening to a heavy drone and gust of whirling winds, above me was this gigantic metal bird — its wings creating a vortex of warm winds. Blaring through a loudspeaker, a lifeguard cautioned me to return to the safe confines of human existence at the shore. I was unafraid of this wide expanse but began to swim back, heeding his warning.

It is always exciting to rummage through little antique shops. There was a certain fervour amidst everyone to step into one particular rather well-advertised shop. But for some obscure reason, I chose to step into a small shop to the left, seemingly all by myself, except for an elderly bespectacled gentleman, overly attentive. In the dim light of one corner of the store, above an old mahogany, carved cupboard stood a statue in isolation, quite lost to the surroundings in the darkness of obscurity. I asked to see it.

Placed gently in my hands, all of 14 inches in size, was the most beautiful statue of the Madonna, revealing herself through a sheath of dust. Wiped of all the dust, she came into her own, moulded of clay from Earth, her hands folded in deep reverence, waves of dark hair textured to one's touch, folds of deep blue and dark rose draping her still and tranquil being.

Her face captured the holy joy of sublimity. A million prayers rested on those lips, and reverie lay behind those gently downcast eyes. Such exalted blessedness and Divine grace emanated from her through the expression of clay in the sculptor's hands. She holds a place of deep reverence in my sacred space, watching over me. I lovingly place roses at her feet and the first flowering Easter lily from my terrace garden.

The Mother of God always manifested in my heart emotions of bravery, deep sympathy, compassion, tolerance and love. Bravery for watching her son being brutalised by man's bestiality, yet contained in her dignity as a woman She sympathised with the plight of mankind with deep tolerance, feeling compassionately for Mary Magdalene, Jesus's companion. Her mystery wove its own gentle patterns through the weave of life.

Strega, the Magical Woman

'To know how to be reborn into a new life at every moment is
the secret of eternal youth.'

Strega! My serene, gentle Italian friend would address me affectionately at times, which is Italian for 'witch'. I guess he knew what was
to unfold, for he had silently watched me float into the depths of
meditation on the lush banks of the placid lake in the Alps.

Talking about *karmic* connections and coincidences? On a flight from
Amsterdam to New Delhi, I was kept awake by the constant attentive
glances of a man sitting diagonally across from me. There was no
exchange of words, but his gaze was unnerving.

He never gave up and on landing, broke the silence and verbally
registered his presence. We met up during his seven-week stay in the
city and found out we both shared the same day, date and year of being
born. A *karmic* connection was there and took us into other regions. He
was a kind soul of gentle demeanour, with a childlike laughter, down
to Earth and thoughtful.

On the day of his return to Torino, he placed in my hand a token of
bonding, a dictionary with translations between *Inglese-Italiano*, which
bore his thumb imprint in blue ink. And on each of the 703 pages, he had
written, '*Ti AMO*'. His eyes brimmed with tears as he placed a bunch of
red roses in my fold. His silence spoke of feelings from another lifetime.

Within a few months, I followed on a trail of gentleness and loving kindness to sunny Italy. Flying into Torino, stepping into the cockpit, I took pictures of the setting Sun in the dusky sultriness of the beautiful Alps. Summertime is simply Nature's expression of beatitude. The pilot and KLM stewardesses found my story right out of a soap opera, wishing me happiness during my sojourn.

We met, both ablush with life's madness, and he drove me into the higher altitudes of the mountain ranges, mostly in nervous silence. Placing a tiny translator into my hands gently, he said, "Relax, Shambhavi, no need to be *nervosa*." There were strains of nervousness. He explained that he had decided on the mountains because he realised the effect they had on my soul. Yes, the mountains always make me feel tranquil.

The vast still waters of the lake sent ripples through my mind, calming my being, sensing a great beauty, peace and joy. I seemed to have been there in an earlier time for sure. Walking to the edge of the water and sitting down on a bed of soft grass strewn with myriad white and yellow flowers, I floated into an expanse of 'no mind', losing myself in meditation. I stayed in this reverie for over two-and-a-half hours, and came to realise Antonio, as was his name, was watching me silently, rather patiently with a smile playing on his lips through the depths of his amber eyes. Sometimes coherence needs no language for expression. The soul reaches out from an earlier lifetime.

On an evening in Rome, I found myself with a childlike fervour, chucking coins into the fountain of Trevi, wishing for happiness. Strolling the cobbled lanes in the vastness of history's shadows, playing hide and seek, I was in deep love and gratitude with the Universe and my life. This was a transient phase for me. The break up of my marriage vows had taken its toll on both of us, I guess. We searched for happiness elsewhere. My self-esteem was at a low ebb; I wanted reassurance to experience the magic of love and warmth, the gentle touch invoking the deep call of my inert femininity.

A new woman seemed to be evolving in her wild search for the unknown, grasping a new-found freedom, experiencing a childlike spirit, the womanly energies of youth, throwing her arms open to the abundance of the Universe. The passionate energies of a zillion flowering sunflowers seem to reciprocate her inner zest.

Yet the callings of the spiritual quest laid to rest my soul. Having met Swami Swarupananda of the Chinnmaya Mission in London, his eyes sought me out and placed in my hands a beautiful book on the experiences of his guru, Swami Chinnmayananda. I sat by the river flowing by my apartment in Torino and taking in the experiences of *sadhakas* all over the world in his book. Time would fly by without my sensing the ticking hands of the watch on my wrist.

I had thrown myself into the fervishness of the world of designing textiles, experiencing the headiness of success; living part-time in New York, creating home fashions for famous design houses, walking down the streets of Manhattan, basking in the womanly pride of watching my designs in window displays and *Vogue* pages. It was madness, a *nasha*, intoxication, till a Thanksgiving dinner brought about a new awareness in my life, slowing the pace down, questioning my very existence.

Miracles — Trail-blazers of Higher Dimensions

The wonders of modern science through its advanced technologies are merely a mechanical channelling of certain outer aspects of the secret powers of the Universe. These secrets are fully accessible through direct inner knowledge in a holistic and creative manner for those who know the yogic art of concentration. The universal consciousness interconnects all things on mental, physical, spiritual, individual and cosmic levels. Men and women who can access its higher dimensions are able to perform metaphysical acts which in the layman's under-standing, are miracles. They are simply following out the secret fabric of the Universe and moving energies along less used or more subtle channels. Through the long course of history, up to the present we come across special individuals empowered to perform such miracles as clairvoyance, telepathy, materialisation, and spontaneous healing.

Perhaps in the mythological past there were beings that in the purity of their innate superconsciousness had a natural ability to access such higher powers. Quite possibly mankind, after enduring the rigours of this *kaliyuga,* may once again regain some of these inner faculties. Today we are blind to these forces and even doubt their existence.

In Vedic thought, each *yuga* or 'world-age' is determined according to varying planetary and solar cycles, bringing to life on Earth different types of cosmic energies and consequent types of evolution and experience. The Earth's geology, flora and fauna change during each *yuga*, reflecting other dimensional connections and parallel worlds, such as is speculated about in science fiction and mythology. In this regard, one could say that the different *yugas* are just different phases of the same experience and can be known simultaneously as different layers of the same life.

Living in the *kaliyuga*, the Dark Age, does not mean that we must all shower dark forces onto ourselves. But reflecting its materialistic mindset, most of us see working with the Divine powers merely as a means to acquire some personal advantage or to undermine our opponents with the help of these 'magical' forces. Only a person with a truly spiritual understanding will use these powers for the betterment of mankind at large. Wise men and women had to guard this secret knowledge to prevent its abuse and misuse by such people.

If we are sensitive to the Divine intent in our lives, we open ourselves to the blessings of the cosmic energies in Nature and remain in harmony with the greater Universe and all its higher dimensions. These were my 'miracles' — the *darshan* of the Mother Goddesses and other deities, telepathic transfers, and healing forces unfolding through me. Such miracles were not dramatic, outer displays of magic but had the inner effect to transform my life from the mundane to the sacred. They helped me understand the miraculous nature of life that we awaken to every day, if we awaken with awareness.

Shakti Samaya: Coming Together with Shakti

'Shiva is within Shakti and Shakti is within Shiva. When Shakti is
unmanifest, Shiva is Absolute and alone. When Shakti is in a state of
becoming, Shiva appears like the Creator.'

Love and seduction permeate the mythology of the goddess, for the
truly blossomed woman is an inexhaustible fountain of sensuous,
magical, tender emotions that transform the heart. The *Tantrika*, the
woman practicing *Tantra*, is the initiator, the birth-giver, and the evoker
of pleasure, kind and compassionate. As the object of the five senses,
she is endowed with the Divine form. In *Tantra*, her entire being is
sacred. The mother archetype is a very important reflection of the
woman's need to provide love, protection and nurturing to her loved
ones. There seems to be a deep longing in each of us to return to the
comfort and bliss within the womb.

The woman's capacity for sexual love is greater than a man's. Out
of a fear of not being able to fulfil this, men have repressed woman's
sexuality, so that most women live without fully experiencing it. Sexual
experience includes the whole spectrum of human emotions and the
play of all the senses. It is love, passion, frolic, a meditation, a prayer
and an offering that can take one to great spiritual heights. A woman
can truly experience this potential, for love to her is unconditional and
comes from her innermost core. Her sexuality is in totality, completely
involving her body, mind and soul.

The sanctity of womanhood down the ages has been defiled, making many a woman manipulative in order to survive. This defilement of womanhood has corrupted society and tainted our very existence. The future of a loving and nurturing social order depends upon allowing women to discover, realise and experience their innocence all over again, secure in the protection of their own hearth and home.

Sexuality lies at the root of life, and we can never learn reverence for life until we learn to respect it. Violence and crudeness in the form of sexual pleasure destroys both men and women alike. Truly the abuse of women is the abuse of the Mother Goddess. As long as the girl child and woman are subjected to violence, trauma or rape at home or in the outer world as a result of crime or war, the very potential of the human family to create a peaceful world can never be realised. That *shakti* is necessary to nourish and support our social order and, if violated, cannot do its work.

Yogini, the Enlightened Woman

'*Aham prema.*'
(I am Divine love.)

In the *Bhavani Nama Sahasra* (Thousand Names of the Goddess Bhavani), Pandit Jankinath Kaul has beautifully explained a *yogini* thus: "A *yogini* is one who is possessed of magical powers." *Para shakti,* the supreme power, in the form of Durga is given the name Yogini. She assumes various forms and takes on different Divine energies to maintain harmony in the Universe, to combat evil and uphold the good. A woman who gains a transcendental state in *sadhana* comes back as a celestial *yogini* or Bhairavi, a female adept at yoga. She carries the energy of Durga within her.

A true *yogini* is an enlightened woman with exuberant passion, spiritual powers and deep insight. *Yoginis* convey a sense of freedom, a sheer mastery in whatever they do. With their compelling gazes, they can hypnotise even a great *yogi* and are capable of changing their shapes at will. *Tantric* scholars have written about *yoginis* as independent, outspoken, forthright women with a gracefulness of spirit. Without them, yoga can fail in its purpose and remain sterile.

Shakta texts honour both women and the Earth alike as sources of energy, vitality, physical and spiritual well-being. Noting this analogy between a *yogini* and the Earth, an 11th-century Tibetan *Cakrasamvara* commentary states: "Having recognised a *yogini* who will delight and transmit energy and power to him, and feeling passionately attracted to her, if the male aspirant does not worship that *yogini*, she will not bless the yogi, and spiritual attainments will not arise." Miranda Shaw's book, *Passionate Enlightenment*, which was introduced to me by Lokesh Chandraji, first exposed the world of the *yogini* to me from a Buddhist perspective.

In Hindu thought, the *yogini* represents the *yoga shakti* herself, the *kundalini*, as well as the resident powers of female deities of the different *chakras*. The *yogini* possesses the power of yoga herself and can awaken that in others, not only generally but at any point or place in the body or mind. A man's ability to achieve the higher states of yoga can be facilitated by his association with such a female companion who reflects this energy.

Just as a goddess blesses and benefits her devotees, and the *shakti* vivifies all biological, cultural, and religious practices, so a woman can channel this life-force or spiritual energy to her consort-devotee. A woman is no more depleted by providing this spiritual nourishment than a mother by nursing her child. In fact, it causes deeper energies to well up from within her.

This spiritual energy is not something that a man can extract or take from a *yogini* at will. She chooses when and on whom to bestow her blessings. Her ability to enhance a man's spiritual development depends upon her innate divinity as awakened and brought to fruition by her own yogic practices, which include envisioning herself in the forms of various goddesses and investing herself with their appearances and ornaments, tender and wrathful expressions, and supernatural powers for liberating beings. By conferring energy and grace upon a man — blessing or empowering him — she is not weakening herself but rather sharing her energy voluntarily with one who has won her favour by meeting the various requirements that she may impose.

Such a relationship is parallel to human-Divine relationships insofar as the deity is the benefactor and the human devotee, the beneficiary. Although the deity may derive some gratification from the relationship, the devotee has much more to gain than does the sovereign object of his devotion. What supplicants ultimately want from their deity is supreme deliverance or liberation, and this is what male *Tantrics* should seek to gain from their relationships with spiritual women. *Tantric* texts reiterate that a man cannot gain enlightenment without respecting women and allying himself inwardly with a woman. The woman's beneficence is a gracious, yet voluntary response to her devotee's supplication, homage and worship.

The goddess is a great *yogini*, devoted to Shiva, yet matching His powers. She is the embodiment of pure energy, the mother and a matrix of all manifestations, the source of all time, space and creation. As they practiced yoga together, Shakti accepted Shiva as her guru, and He taught her the ways of transcendent being to guide her to her ultimate liberation. Shiva in turn also accepted Shakti as His guru, and she initiated Him into His ultimate liberation by putting Him in touch with the supreme power of consciousness.

Goddess Chhinnamasta, the deity who cuts off her own head, symbolises the great *yogini*, the wonderful consciousness beyond the mind. She represents the opened third eye from which flashes forth the lightning of direct perception that destroys all duality and negativity. She is the *yoga shakti* or power of yoga in its most dramatic action of granting enlightenment. Hence, she is also known as Vajra Yogini. The *vajra* is the supreme lightning force of the inner self.

Chhinnamasta is the *Para Dakini*, the supreme or foremost of the *dakinis*, the attendant goddesses on the yogic path, who are the *yoginis* as the powers of the *chakras*. *Sadhakas* seeking the path of occult or yogic powers should worship her, as reiterated by David Frawley in his book *Tantric Yoga and the Wisdom Goddesses*, invoking her through the *mantra* based on her name as Vajra Vairochani. This facilitates all inner transformations in a dramatic way.

The *yogini* is also Bhairavi or the Goddess of Fire below in the *muladhara* or root *chakra*. It is she who becomes Chhinnamasta as she reaches the third eye and opens the crown *chakra* beyond. Her blood is light that illumines everything.

Mary Magdalene was such a *yogini*, manifesting her *shakti* through the flow of light from her heart and soul. Her Divine love was unconditional and independent of external situations and dogmas. Yet Divine love is not limited to the ascetic. In my understanding of *Tantra*, if two spiritually evolved beings come together in unconditional love, they also can create an energy field that is most positive and rare, exuding high vibrational levels of peace and love into the Universe.

The ancient cultures of Egypt, Greece, Tibet and India have esoteric traditions glorifying the initiatory power of the woman. She is considered to be the high priestess, who unfolds all higher knowledge and powers for us. She is Sophia, the source and font of wisdom or *prajna*, the deepest insight into the nature of things. *Tantric* teachings stress the importance of physical beauty in a companion but only to initially stimulate and then elevate passion from the sensual to the spiritual plane. The beauty of the soul surpasses physical beauty.

The 'initiatory' power of woman is tremendous, providing the force of passion that is necessary for developing experiential mysticism. By sharing the secrets of love, a woman can bestow transcendental power on her lover. The highest form of *shakti* is the direct expression of the wisdom-energy she releases, creating a joyful transformation. A woman can initiate her partner into such mystical experiences through trust, surrender to higher ideals and spontaneity. It is the goddess within each woman who really initiates.

To be a *yogini* is the highest spiritual goal for all women. It is the way to become one with the goddess within and to bring her out in expression to uplift the world that is really her creation. Yet it is not an outer appearance but a state of inner energy and ecstasy that makes the *yogini*. She cannot be manipulated, defined or even ever entirely known.

Yogini, the Enlightened Woman

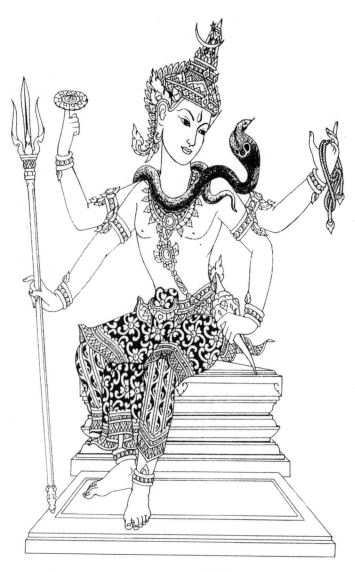

Siddhas, Yogis and *Sadhakas*

Mahavatar Babaji

'Siddhah svatantrabhavah.'
- Siva Sutra 3.13
(A *siddha* lives in total freedom.)

Who are the *siddhas*? They are the ancient and ever-present supreme masters of *yoga*, those who have achieved a mastery over the mind and who manifest various *siddhis*, yogic miraculous powers. The Sanskrit term translates as someone who has merged his sense of individuality into the supreme consciousness of God. The *Shiva Purana* tells us a great deal about the *siddhas*.

The history of the *siddha* tradition goes back to Shiva's initiation of his consort Parvati into the secrets of yoga in the Himalayas. Shiva Yogeshwar, the great Lord of Yoga, later initiated many great *siddhas* like Gorakhnath and Matsendranath from whom most *siddha* lineages arise.

Many revered *sadhakas* mentioned to me the existence of the immortal Mahavatar Babaji, also known as Shiva Baba, Nagaraj and Kriya Babaji. One of them had his *darshan*. I had no idea what his physical features were. My inner being began to want to know more about Babaji. As a young woman I had read about him in the *Autobiography of a Yogi*. My curiosity led me to delve through the pages of Paramhansa Yogananda's experiences over and again.

My favourite little bookshop in Rishikesh, the Sivananda Emporium, always held something of interest for me. I would look forward to spending time there and chatting with the retired colonel who ran the store. And there I had my first glimpse of Babaji, his strength and magnanimity in a supreme state of enlightenment staring at me through the stillness of his being from the picture. He seemed to capture the 'youth of 16 summers', for they say his body had not aged since the age of 16. Pristine, powerful, an intense aura of silence surrounds him.

More people came into my life closely associated with Babaji. I saw the most beautiful statue of Babaji in a *sadhaka*'s place, my friend Girijesh, who threw immense light on Babaji. I guess this was my time to turn to Babaji for his blessings. Babaji spoke, "Take one step towards me, and I'll take 10 towards you."

Babaji is a great master of *Kriya Yoga*, living mysteriously even today in the Himalayas. He had mastered 'death' and attained a supreme state of enlightenment. He was reputed to be a guru of Adi Shankaracharya. In a poem, he writes about Dakshinamurti, whom some identify with Babaji, as a youthful teacher seated under a banyan tree surrounded by aged disciples. Babaji instructs his disciples through silence, which in itself says a lot about the spiritual master. Sri Yukteshwar, the guru of Yogananda, talked of Babaji as a *maha avatar*, a great *avatar*, the Sanskrit word for 'incarnation of the godhead in human form'.

According to one tradition, Babaji made a long pilgrimage to Badrinath, the ancient temple of Lord Vishnu in the form of Badrinarayan. He spent many months practicing the yogic methods taught to him by his gurus and eventually entered a state of *samadhi*, in which the divinity directly descends and transforms the spiritual, intellectual, mental, vital and physical body of a person. Babaji's physical body ceased to age and shone with a golden lustre of divinity. Babaji, since attaining this state, assists humanity in the quest for God-realisation. He has remained in his physical body, visible to only *sadhakas* in this physical world when he initiates them in silence.

The 'silence' about him I learned to appreciate much later. Earlier, during my *sadhana*, I talked to him, sometimes deeply upset as to why he sat there in stoic silence and never reached out to me in my quest for guidance. I would continue my *sadhana* hoping that he would appear. I had always been very vocal in my relationship with my deities, whether in expressing joy or deep anguish. I always took this liberty with Babaji as well.

Driving through the Himalayas, on my way to Kedarnath, the ancient shrine of Lord Shiva, I was lulled into a placid mood as I watched the emerald waters of the beautiful River Ganga winding through the valley off the road. The rays of the warm afternoon Sun comforted me in the early autumn. My mind seemed to experience the zeal of divine joy.

Then suddenly Maha Avatar Babaji's torso appeared in front of me in the car. I sat forward as I had lost my breath. His face was filled with a serene youthfulness, his dark eyes smouldering; his hair seemed fuller than in pictures and was flowing down to his shoulders. The silence, stoic yet powerful, was all pervasive around me. A deep flush swept over my being, leaving me with a gentle tremulous feeling. I slowly regained my breath and Babaji receded into the space in front of me. I so much wanted him to stay with me longer.

This was a deep supernatural experience for me and left me in a wondrous daze. I had no time to ponder the reasons for his *darshan*, the culmination of a yearning of several years. In my heart I was sure this was only the beginning; there was more to come my way.

Surya Yogi

'O Lord and essence of light, lead me from the unreal to the real
from the darkness to light, from death to immortality.'
–*Brihadaranyaka Upanishad.*

His gentleness in white cotton flowing robes breezed into the room; his face shone with warmth, his eyes piercingly dark. 'Let there be light,' Suryaswami Acharya Jowel K. Gopinath's silence seemed to be saying! 'We are going to rule the world 12 years from now,' All of his tall, dark, shyly handsome being quietly stating, 'Yes, me and the followers of the Sun.'

We were gathered at my friend Gita's home, in her basement that was named Moonbeam. On a Sunday she had cajoled me to come and listen to the yogi speak. Sitting at the back, I was placed in the line of his direct gaze. His eyes pierced my depths, stirring a deeper feeling. For the first time I saw a most beautiful aura around a person; bright white on all sides with a violet halo around his head, quite amazingly holding my attention.

After the discourse, walking up close to him, he looked deeply into my eyes and smilingly placed a bright red apple in my hands before whispering very gently, "Great things are going to happen with you; be brave." I felt my eyes brimming and I smiled back at him and mentioned the aura I had seen surrounding him. He reminded me so much of Jesus in his gentle demeanour and compassionate aura. "Come to Mumbai and meet me !" he said.

Suryaswami's search began at the age of seven. He stopped his formal education after the tenth grade and enrolled himself in an *ashram* in Kerala, where he studied philosophy, astrology, astronomy, ayurveda and yoga. He soon outgrew the rigidity and restrictions of the *ashram* and set off in search of more universal truths in the countryside and the Himalayas. He recalls how he studied the science of solar energy after meeting *sadhus* in the bitter cold caves of the Himalayas who survived only on the energy that they derived from the Sun. Out of these studies and experiences, he invented his *Surya Yoga*.

His philosophy, called *Surya Yoga*, emphasises God as an energy, force and spiritual power that guides us to find the answer to the most pertinent of all questions, 'Who am I?' And this search needs a medium to help us unravel the answers. The medium can be anything, a guru, a friend, or even an animal. Being one with Nature, especially with the Sun, plays an important role in unfolding this experience. In *Surya Yoga*, he explains, a new way of life and a meditation technique through which one takes energy from the Sun and uses it to open the higher faculties within us. It results in a simple quest for the self, which is the inner Sun in the hearts of all beings.

The king of the solar system, the Sun, sets in motion the flow of *dharma*, the cosmic law. As per Vedic scriptures, the Sun is the dwelling place of the *rishis* and the *mantras*. The brilliant, effulgent mass visible with the naked eye is only the Sun's physical existence The Sun's consciousness is represented by a warrior-king riding his chariot, driven by seven horses that represent the seven rays of light and their energising powers.

According to *Tantra*, Kamala, the Lotus Goddess of Delight, is worshipped by realising the Divine beauty manifest in the world of Nature. This occurs by meditating upon the rays of the Sun, not as mere material forces but as powers of Divine light and life. Through the rays of the Sun, we are touched by Divine grace and enlightenment. We gain access to all the realms and powers of light externally and internally.

The *Aitareya Upanishad* enlightens us with the statement: "Fire becoming speech, entered the mouth. Air becoming breath, entered the nostrils and the Sun becoming sight, entered the eyes..." The Sun is the supreme eye and grants us all higher powers of perception.

To this omnipotent Lord Surya Narayana, the Sun-god, I offer water and obeisance with *mantras* every morning. Everything originates from the Sun, for he is the soul of the Universe, the king of the sky, and the ruler of all that falls between the Earth and the celestial regions. The Lord of the eastern direction, he is the cause of the day and the giver of bliss. The Sun rules both the sign Leo and the day of Sunday. Time has no reckoning without the Sun and there can be no poetic meters, seasons or rhythm in the world, without his movement.

A Seed is Sown

'In this net it's not just the strings that count
but also the air that escapes through the mesh.'
- Zen poem

On a Sun-drenched afternoon during the winter months I was escorted to a luncheon by a very sensitive, intelligent Frenchman, deeply ingrained in philosophy and mythology, Come Carpentier. I grew to share a very special relationship with him — one of deep friendship, trust and a great sense of humour sheathed with barbs of mischievous innuendos.

The mystery and magic of India drew Come Carpentier into its fold at a very young age, when he used to visit with his father , the late Jean A. Carpentier, a French writer and orientalist in the mid-70s and realised the philosophy and culture of India through the Theosophical Society and Rukmini Arundale. He delved into the studies of Sanskrit, Vedantic philosophy and Carnatic music and dance, opening up to its deeper mystic revelations.

The farmhouse of J.C. Kapoor was wonderful and peaceful, with peacocks strutting around unaware of us around the Surya kund, a great outdoor *yantra* designed for special gatherings. It turned out to be a very interesting afternoon and I met two beautiful dynamic women, Rita and Prem, fighting ardently for a peaceful world.

Then I noticed sitting silently in the centre, right across me was gentleman, dressed in a *dhoti kurta*, a shawl wrapped around his shoulders, observing everyone more than participating in the ensuing conversations. This, I soon learned, was the great scholar, Lokesh Chandra.

Towards the end of the evening when we began to bid our adieus, Lokeshji, who had not spoken to me directly, enquired from my French friend about me and asked if I had practiced or studied *Tantra*. In India, scholars are shy to approach women. I was then introduced to him but without making much conversation. Yet within the next few days I was asked to contact him.

Prof. Lokesh Chandra unravelled the great tradition of art and philosophy in Buddhism through his many distinguished works. He revolutionised our modern understanding of the culture of Asia, as he opened up unknown texts, facts and evaluations in his profound writings. A man of discipline, he adhered to a strict schedule with a clockwork precision. He invited me to visit him at his home, where with deep regard and affection as well as with much humour and mirth, he shared his inner knowledge and wisdom with me.

The first time ushering myself in, quite intimidated with his repertoire of knowledge, I sat down across the table from him, in a spartan high ceiling office. He began the conversation with a real dressing down of *sadhakas*. "You *bhaktas* are in another world, one of make-believe, devotion and hallucinations. We scholars believe in none of this. Ours is a world of knowledge based on facts."

Having listened to his tirade for over half an hour, I shyly replied, "Lokeshji may I share one of my very recent experiences with you? A few days ago during my *sadhana*, I had my head severed from my body in one clean sweep, without a single drop of blood being shed in the process. There was no fear at all within me. Hundreds of owls were swooning around me. So clearly were they visible that I could see their yellowish, sprightly eyes darting in all directions, and their feathers marked beautifully in shades of brown and black. The whole experience was mesmerising." All of this said while Lokeshji was watching me intently, staring me straight in the eyes. I paused, for with the reminiscing of the experience my body was beginning to feel the vibrations, and I gave myself time to settle back into the present moment.

Very gently he spoke, "You are a *yogini* in this life."

I was taken aback, and playfully retorted, "Lokeshji, what makes you believe me? Maybe this is just my hallucination. The *yogini* has very deep meanings, and you are the master of all the knowledge." He then guided me to his library and showed me some books, which he wanted me to read. We grew to respect one other and we met often.

In Hindu, Greek and Roman mythology, the owl symbolises great wisdom and intelligence because of its ability to presage events. The owl is the penetrator of the darkness. It is the symbol of the feminine, the Moon and the night, being a bird of magic and darkness, of prophecy and wisdom. Symbolically, the owl remains as a powerful metaphor for inner wisdom and the regenerative powers of the feminine principle. The pre-historic Mother Goddess was often depicted as a woman with the head of an owl.

Traditionally, the owl is the *vahana*, vehicle of the Goddess Lakshmi. When the depth of darkness is visible, only *astha,* faith will unfold the way in the form of the owl. Birds are complex dream symbols. Flying birds represent movement, symbolising physical or mental freedom. Moreover, flying birds in colour are auspicious omens. Birds also symbolise the higher self. The owl seemed to have come into my fold as a part of my life, or was it the form of *sadhana* I was initiating. They appear frequently for me.

One afternoon, I sailed into Lokeshji's workplace and became intoxicated by the strong aroma of the 'Haar Shringar' blossoms, tiny white flowers with a magical inner orange colour that were placed in his room. So powerful was the scent it sent me reeling to another intoxicating experience — a visit to the Nizamuddin Dargah on a full Moon night, having gone to listen to the *qawwals*, passionate renditions to Allah by Sufi saints. Walking down narrow lanes, I was surrounded on either side by shops laden with the *desi gulab,* the Indian rose with an intoxicating fragrance, usually grown for distilling rose water, and used as offerings.

Masha Allah! Such intoxication, adding to the passionate renditions of *qawwalis* and the *nasha* of the full Moon used to send my mind reeling. Jelaluddin Rumi's beautiful poetry would flow through my mind, *"The minute I heard my first love story I started looking for you, not knowing how blind that was. Lovers don't finally meet somewhere; they're in each other all along. "*

That afternoon over a cup of *chai* and several exchanges of experiences and knowledge, Lokeshji prodded me to express myself in a book. I was hesitant and shy of sharing my experiences as they certainly were unusual and so far had been kept very close to my heart. Though I used to write them down under the dates in a small diary, which was kept in my sacred space, I had not published them anywhere to that point.

He made me realise how helpful such a book might be in encouraging other *sadhakas*, who might not have had any guidance or guru, and were probably as unsure and lost as I may have felt at times. Agreeing to give the project a thought in the future, while walking out he placed in my hands the huge ceramic hand painted bowl filled with the '*Haar Shringar* ' flowers. I felt myself blushing with shyness and he wouldn't allow me to refuse. My drive home was filled with the darkly sweet aroma of the flowers.

One evening, I accompanied him to the Japanese embassy, where he was speaking on the occasion of a book being released. The book was written to commemorate the deep thoughts of Hajime Naka Murra, the guru to the present Emperor of Japan, a teacher that Lokeshji had been closely associated with during his lifetime. It was an evening that began to draw me into the Buddhist *Tantra*. My earlier knowledge of Buddhism was limited to the works of the gentle Vietnamese monk, Tich Nhat Hanh, a few books written by the Dalai Lama and my own personal initiations into Green Tara and Avalokiteshvara.

Lokeshji was never a man of social flippancies, though he had a great sense of dry humour. He walked through the door with a most beautiful bouquet of roses, the deepest shades of flushed pink, which were given to him as a gesture of respect from the ambassador. A young lady student of his requested a single rose from the bouquet. 'No!' was his brusque reply. Later when we sat together in the car to drive back, he reached out, placing the pink roses into my hands, 'This is for you, the Nagakanya!' I was happy to be lost in the darkness of the night for I felt a deep pink flush through my face, "*Shukriya*."

My most unexpected blessing from him came in the guise of arranging a meeting with Pandit Vamadeva Shastri, Dr David Frawley. Having mentioned his book on the Wisdom Goddesses in a conversation, Lokeshji said that he knew the author and I coerced Lokeshji into writing him. In the typical manner of Lokeshji, he addressed a letter with just a "David Frawley, Santa Fe, New Mexico"! Strangely, the letter did reach its destination and we received a confirmation mentioning of his plans to soon visit New Delhi.

Mystical are the creations; Vishvakarma, the celestial architect, weaving into the cosmic web the threads of our life.

The Falcon Takes its Flight

'All this in the beginning was Brahman. That knew itself as
'I am Brahman'.
Therefore, it became everything. Whoever among the gods
or among *rishis* and mortals
awakens to this truth also becomes that. Seeing that,
the Rishi Vamadeva proclaimed,
'I was Manu and I became the Sun'.'
-- *Brihadaranyaka Upanishad*

I was looking forward to meeting Pandit Vamadeva Shastri,
(Dr David Frawley), having read several of his many books. My
favourite was *Tantric Yoga and the Wisdom Goddesses*, a book I referred
to for information on Her various forms, every time She appeared to
me and remained by my bedside at all times. Through the years
of intense pondering on the energies of the *devis*, my passionate
flow and the author's *shakti* seemed to form an amalgamation of *Tantric*
magic permeating my life.

As a *sadhaka*, surely I was in awe of him, a man who went into the
depths of Vedantic scriptures, imbibing them into his own life, literally
making the Vedantic tradition a way of life. There was a quickening in
my pulse rate as I stepped into the beautiful estate of B.M. Thapar and
his ever so gracious lady. Peaceful vibrations emanated from the various
statues of Lord Buddha, an abundance of white and pale aubergine-
hued lilies filling the air with their intoxicating aroma. The morning
sunshine filled the room with an air of exuberance.

My gaze caught the silhouette of a tall, slim man, the contours of his face shadowed by his beard, the soft gentle look in his far away eyes smiled into a greeting. Vamadeva Shastri was for real; not just a sketched portrait on the back cover of his book. There was a definite twinkle, sparks of a silent fire emanating from the depths of his eyes. His energies would draw my deeper yearnings towards him, catching the glints in his eyes, unconscious of the *lila* that was unfolding, changing the course of my flight on the wings of the great falcon.

Along with Vamadeva, I was fortunate to meet N.S. Rajaram from Bangalore and Dr Hussain Khan from Pakistan. Khan Saab was of a gentle demeanour, though fearless and uncompromising in his spiritual views and practices, head of the transcendental meditation (TM) movement in Pakistan from his home in Peshawar and an advocate in the Supreme Court of Pakistan. Khan was visiting India at Vamadeva's request.

Rajaram was a man of great wit with a quick presence of mind, a scientific background, having been an academic and industrial researcher doing a stint with NASA. Being a historian and having authored the book, *Vedic Aryans and the Origins of Civilisation*, with David Frawley, he could steer the conversation into any field. There was a warm and caring aspect about him, which really held my attention. We kept in touch over the e-mail and he would send me his books to peruse, accompanied by music of the chanting of *mantras*.

Our group conversations trail-blazed from challenging deep-seated religious dogmas, going beyond Rightist and Leftist viewpoints, exposing brutal attacks on Hinduism, distortions of history, ecological imbalances and bringing about world peace and a higher age for humanity. We made a formidable group of some firebrand men and women airing their viewpoints, bringing awareness to the forefront.

Vamadeva drew me into his fold unknowingly and I began seeking guidance from him in my *sadhana*. Here was a man deeply sensitive to the subtle nuances of all the five *tattvas*, the elements, relating to their higher vibrations and in its wake experiencing the *rasa* and the life-force existent in them.

His work spanned the fields of yoga, Ayurveda, *jyotish* (astrology), *Veda* and *Vedanta*, with a special insight how *Veda* and *Tantra* worked together for connecting us with the higher forces of Nature and consciousness. His understanding of Vedic and *Tantric mantras* and deities reflected his contact with the teachings of Ganapati Muni, the great yogi and chief disciple of Ramana Maharshi, about whom a few people know.

Vamadeva seemed to allay my hesitation in invoking Kali more passionately, and I opened my arms to her. There was no more hiding my face under the pillow when I'd sense her presence. Yet I waited patiently for the time when Ma would deem me ready to strike a conversation with her, if ever!

Awakening me to the power of Shakti at Kamakhya in Assam, he gently enforced upon me the need of the hour of transformation, the rebirth of Shambhavi. I decided to offer myself at the feet of Kamakhya or Kamakshi, which was also the place of my birth, as part of a special pilgrimage there.

Vamadeva understood my soul, having looked into the finer nuances of my astrological chart. His personal writings gave my life a new style, a calligraphic flourish to the heights of esoteric delving, with the lightning force of *vidyut shakti*.

My childlike exuberance got the better of me when with his book in hand, I shyly asked him to express his thoughts for me. His pen gave flow to my *sadhana*: "Let the Devi come forth through you, her time has come! Jai Ma!"

Till then my concentration and experience was more with the *rudra* form of the Mother Goddess; Vamadeva gently brought in the flow of *soma*, into my *sadhana*, giving vent to the form of Tripura Sundari, and Rajarajeshwari.

Vamadeva, I learned from him, was the name of a great Vedic *rishi*, seer, of the fourth book of the *Rigveda*, and quoted in a major way in the *Upanishads*. The Vamadevas were the *purohits* of the kingdom of Videha from which Sita came and where the great, enlightened king named Janaka held important meetings of the *rishis* and yogis of India.

Vamadeva was also a name for Indra, the foremost of the Vedic *devatas*, who represents the direct perception of the *purusha*.

I was also aware of Vamadeva as a name of the northern face of Lord Shiva. Yet strangely this Vamadeva was from America, from New Mexico, where I had visited in the past, showing the boundaries of East and West are no more.

'Jai Vamadeva!'

Spiritual Guidance
Shows Me the Way

'Gurur upayah.'
(The guru is the means.)

My first meeting with the gentle, yet powerful *guida spirituale* Ashokji came about when through the curiosity of having heard of his clairvoyant prowess, I ventured to meet him. They say at every phase when one is ready, the teacher will appear to you; there is no point in searching him out. Dressed in the traditional white, with a red border Bengali sari, my trademark large red *sindoor tilak*, *gajras*, the Indian flowers with a sensuous aroma we women adorn our hair with, I sat in silence running my *mantras* through my mind, awaiting his arrival.

I felt his presence before he arrived! A tall, athletic build, *savla* (olive complexion), gentle presence wafted in. I stood up in obeisance and folded my hands in a demure *namaste*. He gestured me to take a seat next to him. For a moment I couldn't have eye contact, and we sat in silence. He shut his eyes and began concentrating. I tried to gather guidance from his divine source, but he opened his eyes, cracked his fingers with a loud sound, and drifted into concentration again. I took it as an indication that he was finding it difficult to break into my psyche.

And then we gazed into each other's eyes and he softly began speaking, "You are searching for red roses, deep pure red roses, *ab kahan milte hain* (where do you find them nowadays). Now we get the beautiful hybrid roses, but they have no *khushboo* (fragrance)." He continued, "I see you visiting a powerful temple where there is an *arati* taking place; several lamps are lit up and there is a small conical-shaped rock formation," and he folded his hands making a mound shape.

"Yes!" I said excitedly. "I am going to Kedarnathji in a few days and the *Shivalingam* there is in the unique formation of a rock in the shape of the hump of a bull. They have a beautiful *arati* where the Maharaji, the head priest lights up a lamp with several flames." My *darshan* at Kedarnath was celestial and divine. I spent a lot of time with the elderly Maharaji, the head priest. On a Monday afternoon, sitting at the Maharajji's feet, he made me a delicious drink of almonds and milk, which I opened my fast with. I finished the drink and got up to wash the glass, but this he wouldn't allow me, taking the glass from my hands and washing it himself. I was embarrassed and realised how very humble these great men are. He showered me with his blessings.

He sent me to spend one night in the temple in meditation. Next evening he led me to the inner sanctity of his *mandir*, where he asked me to pay my respects to Ma Parvati in the form of a beautiful bronze statue. On stepping out, he removed the yellow cloth resting on his shoulders and draped it round my neck, placing a box in my hands. The stainless steel box was filled with *bhasma,* holy ash, used in smearing the forehead and body of Shiva *bhaktas.*

Back home in Delhi, I called on Ashokji to tell him about my experiences at Kedarnath. Before I could begin he spoke, "You have been to a Parvati temple and taken her blessings. And someone gave you a yellow piece of cloth to wear!" I was so taken aback and told him about the Maharajji placing the cloth over my shoulders. Ashokji asked me to wear it during my meditations.

Two of my girlfriends wanted to meet Ashokji for guidance. While Sonia was sitting with him, I overheard him say to her, "Don't cross your *Lakshman rekha*." *Lakshman rekha* is the line Lord Rama's brother Lakhsman drew around Sita, forbidding her to cross the line while he and Rama were away, hence protecting her honour. It is also a protective line used in *Tantric* rites. When Sonia stepped out, I asked her why Ashokji should have said something so strange to her. She burst out laughing, "Goodness, I was looking at him and thinking to myself how good looking he is and what legs." I warned her that he could read the mind! I would tease Ashokji about the *Lakshman rekha*.

He soon came over to my home for dinner, which is rare, and I was touched. I brought him into my sacred space and it was beautiful to watch the Mother Goddess speak through him, giving guidance. His eyes had an other-worldly gaze about them and there'd be a childlike smile playing on his lips; sometimes his voice would alter its tone, "Shiva is wanting to come to you and you are holding back, surrender to him, Shambhavi!"

It was a warm summer's evening when I was given my initiation into his *guru mantra*. Dressed in white, carrying offerings for the master of red roses, fruits and sweetmeats, I sat at his feet listening to him speak. Suddenly, in place of him, I saw a man's face with a grey beard and a white halo superimposed. He was clearly reaching out to me from another dimension, asking me what I really wanted as a boon from Ma. I asked for the boon of a healing touch.

He led me into his temple and through simple rituals blessed me with the *guru mantra*, whispering it into my ear ever so gently, leaving me in silence to contemplate in his revered space. My eyes came to rest on a framed picture; it was the same face I had seen earlier superimposed, being one of his guru's. My questioning never seemed to end.

There were moments when I'd move away into silent modes and would receive loving messages from him, keeping me in his heart and never wanting any hurt to come my way. But I was experiencing a vacuum, a void, which needed to be filled.

The Silent Pharaoh

'And though death may hide me, and the greater silence enfold me,
yet again will I seek your understanding.'
— Kahlil Gibran

At the age of 42, I chanced upon a sensitive, evolved, God-fearing man with extensive knowledge of the traditional Hindu philosophy. MK, having studied design in Europe, had the flair for using both the left and right brain, and with training in traditional *Tantra*, used the mystic sciences to flow into modern designs. We gravitated towards each other in thought and shared our views on life, seemingly finding ourselves caught up in the whirlpools of existence, wanting to free ourselves from the commercial world, weave our dreams around a holistic existence and place the bits of the puzzle together to view the larger picture.

We were disappointed on several occasions when we could not decipher the codes. We desperately wanted to shift to a higher dimension of existence, but found ourselves being drawn back into the web of *maya*. We had to cope with survival in an unscrupulous and harsh commercial world. Our soft approach to life only created more hurdles in our struggle for survival.

A man I deeply learned to love for his principles and gentleness, and yet retained the wispiness of a child was whom I affectionately called, *'Thatha Kaka'*, old crow; he would sharply retort that the crow is

Lord Shani's (Saturn's) *vahana*, vehicle. The crow plays a very significant role in symbolism. 'Kaka' translates as that which is to be driven out.

Curiosity further drove me to a second bout of past-life regressions; there were still answers that I was seeking. I went into a regressed state rather smoothly, entering magnificent open doors gilded with gold work into an opulent marbled space with grand columns. Seated in front was a Pharaoh, short in stature, the unmistakably deeply lined black kohl eyes were of MK! Standing by his side, dressed in white robes upheld at the bosom, was I, with a silver spear piercing my stomach, large and amply rounded carrying an unborn child.

The intense experience was deeply disturbing. I could feel the flow of warm tears streaming down my face and my body began to tremble. I wanted to remove myself from the experience, when suddenly my maternal grandmother appeared before me, followed by the appearance of Bhagwan Ramana Maharshi.

I felt a presence place a tissue in my hand, and a voice gently whispered in my ear if I was okay and wanted to come out of the regression. My grandmother guided me out gently. There was a sense of turbulence deep within and I withdrew into a silence, unable to share my experience with anyone.

Returning home, as if through an acknowledgement of my intuition, MK reached out to me over the phone. He heard my story in silence, and then took a promise from me that I would stop any further regressions. He had a similar experience in Norway, and on his return, one of his students presented him with a picture of the Pharaoh with MK's face superimposed — she had seen him as such.

Despite my promise to him that night, I managed to regress myself again and uncover the truth behind the brutality of the spear going through my womb. The answers explained certain experiences in my relationship with men. I accepted my *karmic* fate with grace.

Over time and space, I had moved on, opening my heart to the manifold blessings of the universe. MK seemed to remain tied down by his own strange value systems between the hearth in the home and fire outside the home, trying bravely to unfold the mystic ways of the surrounding world.

A Clairvoyant Guides Me

'No man can reveal to you aught but that which already lies
half asleep in the dawning of your knowledge.'
- Kahlil Gibran

She held a beautiful, strong presence with powerful energy flowing
from her dark pools of lotus-shaped eyes; a clairvoyant and a healer.
We connected immediately, and over the years I drew to her for comfort
and guidance. She was wonderful, not always telling me what I best
wanted to hear. But we would get lost in time narrating our experiences,
and would have her staff come in to remind us that there were people
waiting for consultations.

She loved to hear about my passion for Shiva and narrated the
experience her father had on his visit to Kedarnath before she was born.
After *darshan*, on his way down hill he came across a huge black *naga*,
a serpent, coming out through the Earth and going in through another
side. Something came over him and he killed the *naga*. But at that very
moment he fell to the ground paralysed. A few *yatris* on their way up
happened to witness this and carried him back all the way to the temple
in a palanquin made from a sheet tied to bamboos. At the temple the
head priest asked him to perform a penance and after finishing the
penance, energy flowed to his legs and he managed to walk down.

On one of my visits, while in an animated conversation with her,
she broke the flow with, "I see Kali behind you; her energies are strongly

there." She was right. Those were the days I had this strong presence in my room, the vibrations of which I was unable to comprehend.

I touched base with her often, or else intuitively she would reach out to me. Most times it was on my birthday in January. This time the night before meeting her, I saw three fig trees growing clearly placed in a row, a statue of Ganapati and a silver Nandi, the powerful yet gentle bull, the vehicle of Lord Shiva. Narrating what I saw, she was taken aback, and hugging her daughter confirmed my vision.

She placed in my hands a most beautiful *yantra* of the *trishul* studded with the *navaratna*, the nine planetary gemstones. The *yantra* carried the most powerful vibrations, and I was to honour its inherent powers over a period of time with beautiful rituals. On the last night of my *sadhana*, I saw an amazing *nagadeva*, serpent-god, rise over my body and with full hooded wonder strike my forehead! I was overawed by its sheer presence.

The Warrior Within

'Stiff and unbending is the principle of death.
Gentle and yielding is the principle of life.'
— Lao Tsu

All life in the cosmos is animated by *Chi*, the 'life-force' or 'vital energy', the universal power. The life-force is central to every culture: *Chi* in Chinese, *Ki* in Japanese, *Diyin* for the Apache Indian, *mana* for the pygmies and *prana* in Sanskrit.

Chi is the cosmic force one senses in Nature, which blends the mind-body power, freely mixing the polarities of *yin and yang*. All life consists of the constant interplay of *yin or ida*, the passive feminine principle and *yang or pingala*, the active masculine principle.

The mysterious power of *Chi* is linked with Taoism and has been tapped for self-healing and self-realisation, nourishing the body and calming the spirit. Only when *Chi* is balanced is it possible to harness it. Both the dynamic *Chi kung* (moving) and passive *Chi kung* (still) should be practiced simultaneously. *Yang* and the *yin chi* reside in the sinews and the marrow and form a protective sheath for the body. The *tan tien* in Chinese or the *hara* in Japanese, the navel centre, is called the 'sea of *Chi*'. Cultivating *Chi* is not merely a technique but a lifelong practice that can set in motion many higher energies and experiences. Its power lies at the root of all martial arts and meditative practices.

The Sensei who initiated me into his fold was truly a silent warrior, slender in body, powerful within; gentle and yielding, yet firm in his conviction. A man of few words, deep in silence, he had a blazing fire in his eyes. I felt a connection with him instantly. There was a passion about him, which gave vent to the stealth and magnetic flow of his movements, powerful almost ballet like in style, scripting a 'meditation in motion'.

I wanted to deeply study this Taoist form and accepted him as my master. *T'ai Chi* opened up an understanding of *prana*, the great cosmic energy. Its subtle but powerful movements extended from stirring up the gentle breeze of the wind to driving up a storm powerful enough to uproot an oak tree, from the gentle ripple of a soft wave to the turbulent ferocity of a tsunami. Such is the play of elements of wind and water, each giving vent to their inner fires of expression, much akin to our human lives.

He was harsh with me in the class, bringing me out of my reverie, goading me to perfection. His strong barbs sometimes were angled at me. But it eventually taught me the art of perfection. At other times he would remain in stoic silence. There was always a dignity and sensitivity in his silence and stillness, a quiet sublime feeling which communicated a deep compassion without expressing a word.

Life became a vibrating, pulsating passion, reflecting a tremendous energy through my *T'ai Chi* movements. With its gentle movements and silent yet powerful touch, it calmed my inner fires. For me, life's nuances were never to be experienced as lukewarm. To reach beyond mediocrity, I created a life of great passion. Whatever I did, I did wholeheartedly — be it writing, designing, loving, meditating or praying. The sacred is discovered not just at the altar in the temple and not just by searching for the extraordinary, but rather by finding the extraordinary even in the ordinary! *T'ai chi* helped me understand this gentle movement of life-energy that can by its persistence eventually overcome anything.

Mahajanji Walks Me through Delhi's Magical Energies

'And he who has deserved to drink from the ocean of life
deserves to fill his cup from your little stream.'
- Kahlil Gibran

My wonderful elderly *sadhaka*-friend gave me a lot of encourage-
ment through extremely trying times. Once a fortnight he would
take me to all the places around Delhi, where he had experienced truly
powerful vibrations. We would spend hours sitting and he would leave
me alone and watch me from a distance. Delhi is vibrating with such
places. On an evening in the rainy season, we walked up to an isolated
Shiva temple, where was a *samadhi* of a *siddha* from Bengal.

One had to climb up the steps through a dense jungle, right in the
midst of the city. The skyline view was mesmeric, with the rays of deep
crimson of the setting Sun illuminating the evening, a balmy breeze
sending a shiver down my spine. I stepped in to pay my obeisance to
my Lord Shiva and was guided to the nearby *samadhi* of Babaji as they
called him.

I stood in silence by the *samadhi*, in a state of 'no mind', for there
were no thoughts at all. Then I heard a distinct voice from the depths of
the *samadhi*, very gentle and soft, and my feet begin gently quivering. I
pulled myself out of the reverie to see if Mahajanji was nearby and lost
my connection with the other world.

Dargahs hold very special blessings for me; I usually resonate with their vibrations. The Mayee Saab Dargah in New Delhi is the place where Nizamuddin Auliya's mother was laid to rest in her *samadhi*. She was a pious heart-warming soul. We spent an evening there, listening to *qawwalis* rendered in the covered, marble verandah, surrounding her *dargah* near the wide girth of an old tree.

I lit a bunch of incense to offer her and silently stood by her side. We must remember the spirit world is propitiated through the sweet aroma of incense. My mind was blank — no thoughts, and no questions, silent moments, when I was awakened from my reverie, hearing the distinct loud knocking, six times, in beats of three! I opened my eyes to view my surroundings and the knocking was clearly coming from inside the *maqbara* — the grave, a deep, hollow resounding sound.

I looked questioningly across at the person standing in front of me and asked him if he could hear the knocking. He stared at me with a bizarre questioning in his eyes. I looked away, searched out Mahajanji and asked him to stand by my side. When I would raise my hand, it would be an indication that the knocking was happening again. The knocking did happen again in a beat of three distinct times, twice over, and I raised my hand. I opened my eyes and looked at him, and he said, "I hear nothing; the message is only meant for you. Take these instances as silent initiations from the other world, the ethereal world."

We spent quiet evenings, most times sitting in silence while taking in the surrounding vibrations, the gentleness of the breeze and the calmness of Nature. Then there were times when I would open up to him and tell him all my experiences. I always knew he would not ridicule them being a *sadhaka* himself with blessings of the revered Swami Muktananda.

Sensing my confusion and the deep quest to decipher these experiences of mine, he gave me the book *Chitshakti Vilas* — a work of illumination, charged with Gurudev's spiritual force. The book wrote about one of Mahajanji's experiences, for after listening to all my 'strange mystic happenings', he felt I was ready to unravel some of them through Gurudev's experiences.

I never looked back at my experiences during *sadhana* as 'strange' any more. They were a culmination of earlier intense *sadhanas* from other lifetimes as well, and with the *anugraha*, blessings, from the higher powers of the Universe. I no more thought of myself as going crazy. I became more passionate in my search for answers, wanting to speak with the goddesses and ask them a million questions, and so I began even more intense spells of prayer and seeking.

There were always distractions from the world I existed in, emotional and financial, a spectrum of insecurities I'd work very hard in dealing with. Realising these were testing times, failing the test, she would appear in another form to lure me back to her! There were times when I would weaken from my worldly pressures and break down at her lotus feet and sob like a child. She would allow me to cry and then this wave of deep love and calm would sweep over me, pacifying my inner being.

I would end up sitting peacefully and smile to myself — this is the play of *maya*. I would wash my face and look at myself in the mirror. There were no traces of a sobbing child-woman. My eyes would be overflowing with compassion and a soft hue shone over my face just as when you offer the goddess your tears, she takes them from you, and will leave no tell-tale marks.

When you offer yourself to her, she will strip you of your ego. Some of her ways seem very harsh, but she will be there at the top of the cliff that she has pushed you to! This has always been my experience with her. There were numerous instances of difficulties, but in the end I would always surrender to her and in the next moment the right person would walk into my life or simply pick up the phone and comfort me.

Sadhakas have beautiful, most unlikely experiences. On a balmy spring afternoon, I dropped in to catch up with Mahajanji. I was at the door without any intimation and he opened the door, saying, "The sweet aroma of roses wafted in and I could sense you were nearby!" I don't use perfumes. "This is the sweet aroma of *bhakti*," as he gently put it.

In a simple *shloka*, 'Ichha shakti Uma Kumari' (Uma is the power of desire), it explains itself. Whatever we desire Parvati, Uma Kumari will fulfil with her *anugraha*, or grace, because hers is the power of Divine will and aspiration. We have the right to only choose the action or make a wish; the fruit or its fulfilment is left to her.

Sitting at my place, exchanging notes on the various aspects of spirituality, Mahajanji decided to share some *mudras* with me that Muktananda Swamiji initiated him in. While experiencing the *mudra*, my senses were lost, practically shut off. A fiery white flame rose up from my *ajna chakra*, the point between the two eyes where the 'third eye' is situated. My body experienced a strange weightlessness and in the centre of my forehead appeared this large eye in a deep blue colour, outlined with grey. From it shone rays of white brilliance all around. I couldn't tell how long I remained in this mystical trance-like state. Coming out of it, Mahajanji insisted that I take a look at myself in the mirror. I felt a sheer flush for what I saw was a deep glow, a soft resonance of calm illuminating radiance.

Sadhana doesn't give one a ticket to the the joy-rides of life; with it are life's silent trials, sufferings in the layman's language, fruits of our earlier *karmas*, some not so sweet! But these were reminders to me of life's bed of roses with the timely pierce of thorns.

Mahajanji suffered a stroke, which left me deeply questioning, 'Why him, a man of prompt schedule and *sattvic* lifestyle?' I sat with him understanding the harsh realities of the play of life. He amazed me with his grasp of the dictates of *karma* and his graceful acceptance of its results. Yet the child in him rose to his lips in an unguarded moment, "Shambhavi, can you request Ma to heal me? She will listen to you. Pray for me to get back on my feet. Send me your healing energy."

I wanted her magic to work for whatever reasons, and placing my hands on his knees, prayed fervently. The knees truly connect us with the energies of life. Weak knees is a loaded phrase for when our energies run low due to internal turbulences or outside forces, our knees give way first, cutting the powerful support line from below.

I sought *mantra* guidance from my Mevlana to strengthen his nervous system. He proposed a Bhairavi *mantra*, not knowing that Bhairavi was also the main goddess Mahanji worshipped. I directed the *mantra* from my heart to his being, guiding him to say the *mantra* with the force of *prana* alongwith some *mudras*.

In a miraculously short span of time, though he was well into his late seventies, he got back on his feet and with his voice and hands made his offering of Bhairavi's *mantra*. *Jai Ma*!

On my return from Kamakhya sometime later, I called in to see him. So filled with joy was he that in a spurt of excitement, he said that I must have been one of the Bhairavis with Shiva, as per *Tantric* traditions. No *Tantric* or *siddha* was ever without a powerful Bhairavi by his side. I was beginning to have my heart trained on my Shiva; it was a matter of time.

Shiva's Energy Draws Me Out

'Om namaha Shivaya'

Shambhu is a most powerful *sadhaka* who I firmly believe Shiva guided me to; a young man with great experience and knowledge, and a singular passionate thirst for Shiva and the Mother Goddesses. Daredevil was he: no fear of the unknown, in expression and deed. I chanced upon him in the most unusual circumstances! There was a gentleman from Sweden who had been trying to meet up with me for over three months, but somehow the meeting wasn't taking place. In those days I had stopped socialising and wasn't meeting anyone.

Eventually before returning to Sweden he called me, saying that since I wouldn't meet up with him, maybe I would be interested in meeting a successful young Indian entrepreneur, all of 33 years of age, who had a deep knowledge of the *Shastras* and the experience to go with it. I can't remember who called first, but our very first conversation lasted for over an hour and a half. It was spellbinding from the word go! He asked me to come and see him and eventually I ended my vow of not socialising and went to meet him. I was casually dressed, black track pants, orange sweatshirt, hair tied back; the only adornment was my trademark, *vibhuti* and *sindoor tilak*.

We sat in silence, in a rather dimly lit office, taking in and sussing out each other's vibrational levels. The room was heavily charged with electrifying currents. My eye caught a beautiful *murti*, a statue of Maha Avatar Babaji, the first I had ever seen, also the first person I'd come across who connected with Babaji. I knew what brought me here. The pieces of the jigsaw puzzle began to fall in place; this would be a strong association and exchange of *spanda*, vibrations!

After looking at me for some time in the eyes, Shambhu softly, yet firmly spoke, "Why are you hiding from the world and camouflaging your beauty? This is not your role to play. Ma has a more vibrant, powerful role for you to play. Come out of this hiding. The next time I meet you, I want to see you the way you are meant to be, looking beautiful. This is the gift of Shiva; you have no right to disrespect this blessing! " He read my mind so brilliantly. I was taken aback. Most certainly I was not under any hypnotic spell, but in a total state of awareness, and he was right.

The next time I met him happened to be a Monday, my day set-aside for Lord Shiva. I take special care to dress up on a Monday, my way of subtly trying to lure Shiva. I fast during the day and in the evening visit a quaint *Navagraha mandir*, temple, to the nine planets. I cherish and look forward to this day of the week. Stepping out after my obeisance to the Lord, I receive a call from Shambhu and decided to stop by his office. I walked in, dressed in my deep red and green Kanjeevaram saree, flowers in my hair, and customary tilak. He walked past me and I drew his attention with a 'hi'. "*Aap*, I never recognised you!" he replied. We sat for hours talking about the ways and manifestations of the Divine.

One Holi, the festival of colours, we began talking about *The Ten Great Wisdom Goddesses*, reading references from David Frawley's book on *Tantric Yoga*. Our conversation carried on non-stop from 10 in the morning till four in the evening, at which time I took a break to shower and have a quick bite before we got drawn into the conversation again till 10.30 in the night; a marathon discourse on *The Mother Goddess* just over the telephone! I learned a lot from him. He was direct to the point, critical and most encouraging with me. My *sadhana* went ahead in leaps and bounds; we would share powerful *mantras*, including some of the most powerful Aghora practices.

Shambhu on our very first meeting mentioned to me that come Navaratri, Ma would appear to me. And she did! He used to affection-ately call me an *Aghori*. I was very keen to perform a *shava sadhana* in the *shamshan*, the cremation grounds. I had become fearless. We

Shiva's Energy Draws Me Out

identified a particular isolated one, and he decided to accompany me but would sit on the periphery, lest my *sadhana* would get disturbed. But the most beautiful guidance came through him. He instructed me to do a simple, intense *sadhana* in my sacred place in a particular manner, to invoke her with a powerful *matangi mantra*. He was confident as a passionate woman *sadhaka* that I would be successful. I was!

He was very sensitive to my thought waves and would sense when I would be deeply disturbed or insecure. The phone would ring and he would reassure me that all would be taken care of. He did take care of me; he wanted nothing to distract me in my *sadhana*. Here was a completely selfless man, with no expectations or demands, at times protecting me like a child; at other times respecting me as an *aghori*. He instilled fearlessness in me. Coming across a beautiful picture of Shiva astride His bull Nandi, dark and daring, absolutely wild, I had a copy made for Shambhu, and had one framed near my bedside as well.

Shambhu became my spiritual friend, guide, and philosopher. I used to tell him of my dream of wanting to be in a beautiful relationship with a man, whom I would totally surrender to. "No ordinary man will be able to take your powerful vibrations. Surrender to Shiva and He will take care of your needs."

One late evening, he came to my home and placed this beautiful *yantra* carved out in gold with gemstones. "Keep this with you tonight and energise it for me; I will come and collect it tomorrow." That night sitting with the *shani yantra* in my hands was magic! Throbbing in my palms, I sat through the dark hours praying into it. The next day at dusk, after the hour had turned dark, he came and asked me to place the *yantra* around his neck, bowed in reverence and touched my feet. Such humility from such a powerful man!

Later a *rudraksha mala* came into my possession, featuring different faced beads in number from one to 14. It had the most amazing vibrations, varying in tones from black to red, three of the beads with Lord Ganpati's trunk, said to be very auspicious. I would wear this every day, allowing its curative and mystical properties to pervade my being. Shambhu just placed the *rudraksha mala* in my hands and said, "These vibrations are befitting to your *sadhana*." No questions would ever be asked. Our lives never crossed certain *rekhas* or parameters.

There was to be a powerful solar eclipse on a Saturday, and a day prior he called me up and asked me to accompany him to select some lapis lazuli beads, setting aside the ones with more powerful vibrations. From a range of *malas*, I selected the most deep, blue lapis lazuli, with golden sparks offsetting the stones. "Select two *malas* and get them strung with a 14 *mukhi* (faced) *rudraksha*, and wear them throughout the hours of the eclipse, while chanting the powerful *mantra japa*."

I went home and prepared to make the two Shani *malas*. They were truly beautiful; I still wear mine. June thirtieth was the eclipse and early morning I sat in *sadhana*. That evening he came home to collect his *mala*. We were to wear them for 40 days, but on the dark night of the 30th, exactly a month later I shared my apprehensions with him about my *mala* going to break soon. The next morning while showering, my *mala* broke and came apart in my hand. I was taken aback and a little nervous, trying to reason why this should have happened.

Stepping out of the house, while in the car, Shambhu called to tell me that his *mala* broke whilst bathing in the morning! It sent a shiver down my spine and I narrated my experience to him. Both our Shani *malas* broke at the same time, in the same circumstances. What coincidence was this?

It was during the 30 days of wearing the Shani *mala*, when Shani Dev appeared to me.

Shiva's Energy Draws Me Out

Shani Dev, the *Karmic* Leveller

'Aum devindra shanisvaraya namah.'
(I bow with deep obeisance to the king of kings, Shani Deva!)

Shani Dev became my Lord to whom I turned to as a seeking child, never in fear but in complete awe. He is the great leveller of *karma*. Little do we understand his benevolent nature. On a most revered Thursday of June, the 19th, of the year 2003, in my deep slumber there appeared the most beautiful white tiger, powerful in its stealth-like motions, fire in its brilliantly burning eyes. There were children playing around me and in a moment of protective instinct I moved all of them from its path and raising my right foot, immobilised its power. The tiger seemed to succumb for a moment taking the form of a tame silent power. From the sheer blue sky, a pure white silken drape floated across, falling gently into my hands.

I awakened from this deep reverie, curious to decipher the meaning of the experience. While reaching into deep thoughts through meditation, I must have drifted off into slumber once again, only to witness the most powerful form of a well-built man appear before me! He gently draped a long, silken, shining cape of the deepest unimaginable hues of purplish-blue over my shoulders. It was extremely vivid and yet I was unable to pinpoint the exact tone of colour! The dramatic effect of the experience brought me back to the waking stage.

The following Sunday of the same week, I got a call from a friend who has a beautiful farm house on the outskirts of Delhi — a serene, magical place with blue lotuses lazing in the still waters of a small pond. Agreeing to spend some time with him, he drove over to bring me to his home. Named Arun, he was a realised *sadhaka* in many ways. Over lunch, we shared our thoughts and suddenly he asked me if I had been to the Shani *dham*, the Saturn temple, which was very near his place.

We soon got into his car and drove over to the *dham*. Alighting from the car, I found myself facing the most imposing statue of Shani Dev, wearing the same colour of cloak that had been placed over my shoulders, during my sleep! I stood rooted for a moment, mesmerised with his aura, when Arun gently beckoned the *purohit* at the *dham* to escort me inside. I found it difficult to take in all the vibrations.

Lord Shani had come into my life for wonderful reasons, as the wheel of *karma* was unfolding.

Recently, on the 13th of January, 2005 on a Thursday, Saturn was as close as it can get to Mother Earth. It was shining at its brightest during that night. Its illustrious rings were also as wide open as they can get, providing a wonderful opportunity to view them.

The Sun, Earth, and Saturn were in direct alignment, an auspicious time for *sadhana*. Forces were pulling me. I set aside my plans for the evening, took a long walk in the lush Lodhi Gardens as the setting Sun highlighted the historical tombs of yesteryears. My *sadhaka*-friend had mentioned to me of the times when his guru, Muktananda would spend time strolling through these gardens, calling them, *tapo bhumi*. The vibrations of the Earth there are very powerful, the ancient trees releasing their energies into the cosmos.

I readied myself for meditation and began by about half past ten, having surrounded myself with the light of my *diya*, heavy incense, and red roses. Darkness prevailed elsewhere. My meditation with *mantra japas* continued well into the early hours of the next dawn. My whole being was experiencing cosmic vibrations; sometimes an overwhelming sensitivity would pervade my body. My bodily heat was beginning to drench me in sweat and midway I had to change into a black gown. I had put on my special Shani *mala*, which I wear when paying obeisance to Shani Dev.

I seemed to be feeling the cosmic rays from Saturn permeate the Earth and my entire being. I fell asleep in the early morning with Saturn's *beej mantra* on my lips, only to wake up shortly after to find my Shani *mala* removed from my neck. I found it lying besides my pillow. There is no way the *mala* could be removed from my neck without having been broken, so I was surprised! I placed the *mala* safely under my pillow and drifted back into slumber. Strangely though, the *tabeez* on a black thread round my neck was broken away and was lying beside me.

My being felt very light, as if all the weight had been drawn out of it. I was asleep on my stomach like a child. And I felt one hand placed on the back of my head and another simultaneously on my back heart *chakra*. My awareness was acute; I could sense the definite touch of a man's hand, rather large, heavy yet soft in its pressure. I awoke and turned my gaze to my left as the presence seemed to be on that side. Calmness swept over me, and moved me into a very deep slumber once again.

As I write this, an immense blush seems to overwhelm me, a light sweat breaking through my body. Such is the intensity of one's dalliance with the higher powers. Was this Shani Dev? My clairvoyant friend threw a different light over my experience. She seemed to think it was Lord Krishna as she had experienced Krishna's touch, which was of a large, heavy hand!

Dr Robert E. Svoboda rendered the deeper insights to the ways of Shani Dev with his narration of the mythic story, *The Greatness of Saturn*. Mythic stories are a powerful form of therapy, since none of us move through life without being touched by Saturn, who personifies time, limitation and the adversities of life. Through my own experiences with life's journey, Shani Dev was not to be feared, but rather, appreciated with a deeper understanding.

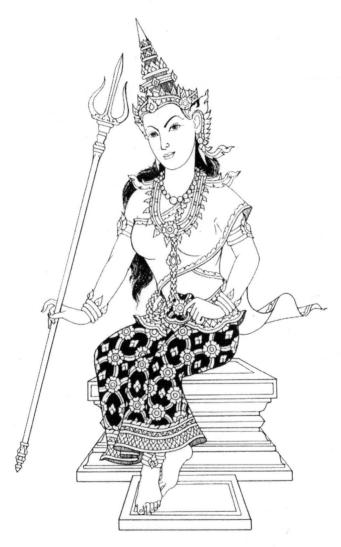

Ma Kali, *Mahaprakriti,*
the Beautiful Goddess

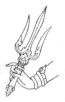

Ma Kali, the Goddess of Light

'Atmano bhairavam rupam bhavayed yas tu purusah tasya mantrah prasiddhyati nityayuktasya sundari.'
- *Siva Sutra (1.137)*
(O Goddess, only he who knows that Shiva is within himself as himself realises the goal of the *mantra*.)

'Kali is the liberator. Kali gives protection to those who know her. Kali is the terrific one, the Destroyer of Time. As the dark *shakti* of Shiva, Kali is space, air, fire, water and earth. Kali performs all the physical needs of Shiva. She is the possessor of the 64 arts and increases the joy of the Lord of creation. Kali is the pure, transcendental *shakti*. Kali is the night of darkness.' - *Kalika Purana*

Parvati, on the highest peak of Mount Meru at the centre of the Universe, implores Lord Shiva to reveal the inner meaning of her mystic form of Kali, the one who is black as the limitless night sky, awesome, fearful, yet compassionate. Shiva explains Kali in the most beautiful, gentlest way as the transcendental peace that follows ecstatic bliss.

In the *Brihad Nila Tantra*, Shiva describes Kali as the primordial one, *Prakriti* (primal Nature), the beautiful woman, the primordial knower, with *kalas* or parts, the fourth (*turiya*), the ultimate Mother, the boon giver, the desirable one, and the lady of heroes. She is

Mahaprakriti, the great substance of everything, Kali, the true form of time, whose great *mantra* of all *mantras* encompasses the ocean of *mantras*. She alone grants all success to a *sadhaka* who wants it. The destroyer of anxiety, giving boons, seated on a corpse, she fulfils all desires and creates all marvels!

The four weeks of January through my 45th birthday brought a strong presence into my bedroom every night. The vibrations of this presence were powerful and persistent. I sensed it was Ma, but couldn't make out her form. Her vibrations were different from those of Ma Tara. I would be like a child and literally hide my face under the pillow on hearing her footsteps, covering my ears to block out the sound of her drawing my attention. For some reason my mind wouldn't allow me to approach her.

The presence became even more aggressive and eventually quite disturbing. At a particular hour every night, to the right side of my bed, I heard a beautiful tinkling sound, like a clink at the rim of a fine Rosenthal flute, along with certain footsteps. It is amazing how each goddess's footsteps differ in sound and vibrations. After a while, she wouldn't even allow me to sleep. In the end, seeking comfort and guidance from my spiritual teacher, I began struggling to find out why I wasn't ready to invoke her.

I went to visit my sister in the Chamba area of the Himalayas in Himachal, where there are many powerful temples. We entered the mountain range at about one in the night, and while everyone was asleep, I began to feel the magic of her vibrations. Each strong vibration would herald the approach of a small temple that we were passing. They were so powerful, lit up with their red lights, that it was as if they were awake, playing their own *lila*. The experience was breathtaking.

One morning, I arranged to meet a temple priest. A young *pundit* walked in and looked strangely at me. After a while, he beckoned me to the side and said that he wanted to speak with me. We sat down in the open verandah overlooking the geese preening themselves in the water. I gently mentioned that I was not keen to know anything about my life or my future. "No," he said, "there is something else I am seeing." I sat patiently and listened, for I needed him to perform a special *havan* I would instruct him to do.

He astral-travelled in his mind to my home in New Delhi, entered my door, then into the kitchen, my mother's bedroom and stepping into the second bedroom, he paused, "I see Ma Kali standing here!" I gently told him that this was my bedroom where I have never invoked her, nor is there any picture of her on my altar. He replied, "But she is here to stay. Once she enters a place, she doesn't leave. Whoever stays in the room and doesn't revere her, will be disturbed because her vibrations are overwhelming." I didn't share with him my experience of the presence I felt over the previous weeks.

It must have been Ma Kali for her vibrations were different from any other I had so far experienced. She was asking for a *bali*, a sacrifice, so we decided we would offer her a white pumpkin, as I am not in favour of animal sacrifice. Yet, strangely, one night several months earlier, I had an amazing vision of the most beautiful large wild fowl, with fiery black and red plumes. It was sacrificed with the powerful force of a single strike and its huge drops of the deep red blood splattered in every direction.

The next evening while driving out into an unknown jungle through a rough road in search of the mystic, Ashiq Allah Dargah, as I stepped out of the car, right at my feet was this huge wild fowl, with the same plumes as in the bird that was sacrificed the previous night, showing me Kali's eternal play of life and death. A shiver went through my being!

To me this was my offering of sacrifice to her; she had made it happen in a vision. Ma always understands her children; their inner natures and their mindsets. She had been preparing for all my future *sadhana*, I am sure. "Ma Kali will always protect you and will only reveal herself to you when you invoke her," the young priest assured me.

Early the next morning, we got a phone call from my niece in Delhi. In tears, she said the cousins had landed into a terrible fight!

Suddenly the young priest's words came to my mind, "Ma Kali would disturb anyone sleeping in my bedroom alone." My son was sleeping there. I rang up my mother and instructed her to move him out of my room!

We sat around the *havan kund* to begin our offerings to Ma Kali. I specifically instructed the *pujari* on how to perform the *havan* with utmost simplicity. Her presence was strong and I began drifting into another world, having to continually keep bringing myself back to the *havan*. The priest must have been quite amused. I was happy with the way things were moving. Her presence was there, at times furiously fanning the flames. This was beyond my expectations.

I See Beautiful Kali

'I bow to the great feminine who
abides in all beings in the form of beauty,'
— Devi Mahatmyam.

Two hours later, we were driving down to Dalhousie to spend some
time at the summer palace of the Maharaja of Chamba. Still in the
throes of being mesmerised by the vibrations of the *havan*, enjoying
the landscape in silence, right there in front of me appeared Ma Kali.
Yes, she had the most gentle, pretty, nubile face in deep hues of blue,
her red tongue protruding from her mouth, her dark eyes moist and
flashing, but not a drop of blood anywhere! I was calm and quite taken
aback by her beautiful soft hues, for at last I received her blessings
with her *darshan*. She suddenly disappeared and the face of a handsome man came in front of me — dark olive in complexion, with a
huge moustache and warm almond-shaped eyes.

Ma Kali appeared to me in her form as youthful, soft, gentle and
beautiful. She had the face of a playful, child-woman. Kali manifests as
beauty at times, the root *kal* behind her name meaning 'to measure',
'apportion' or 'to set in motion', which can translate into beauty as being
'well formed'. Time itself can manifest through rhythm or movement,
creating the dance of the life-force, forming the basis of ethereal beauty.
Beauty is not only loveliness in form. The more we seek beauty of the
inner consciousness, the more we grow beyond the realm of death.

Divine beauty pales every physical aspect of beauty, for when the wistful lotus wilts, it is merely the form that passes away. Ma Kali is the flow of Divine grace from the heart of Lord Shiva, the active power emanating from Him, the life and energy of Shiva, which imparts on each thing in Nature its glow and its resonance.

Still in a mesmerised state, excitedly I shared my 'special *darshan*' with my sister, who was sitting beside me in the car. She looked shocked. To break the silence, I joked with her that probably we were going to meet this man at the palace we were about to visit. We walked into the palace, fairytale-like with wonderful surroundings, and I found myself drawn to the right wing of the building. An oil painting framed on the wall stopped me in my track.

It was the same face of the man who had earlier appeared to me. Silently, with eyes closed, I began to meditate and an owl appeared before me, followed by Lord Ganapati. I was unable to make any connection between the three and I must have looked surprised, as my sister walked up from behind and quietly said, "It's the same face!"

Dharamsala, the residence of the Dalai Lama, has its own special appeal. The people are gentle, the temples projecting their own brand of mysticism, and the market place bustling with tourists seeking *nirvana*. We wound our way through the dark, pine-covered mountainside against the mystical backdrop of the snow-capped Dhauladhar mountain range. An interesting image began appearing before me, taking the form of a *Shivalinga* standing on a silver plate, decorated with intricate work.

We got busy with the market place and then decided to visit the ancient shrine of Bhagsunath. Climbing the steps into a quaint little courtyard filled me with a certain curiosity and, as if guided, I came to the *Shivalinga*. It was of a dark stone slightly lowered with intricately worked silver surrounding it, the same as had appeared in my vision! A quiver went through me; my psychic powers were getting activated. At moments like these I usually withdraw into silence and want to move away from the crowd and remain in isolation, but there are always constraints with friends around.

Driving through the fertile Kangra valley of Himachal Pradesh, Nature unfolded the awe of the Universe, green fields with an abundance of flowers, the snow-capped mountains majestically overlooking the vales, and the azure skies showering us with blessings. There was a song on my lips and a dream in my heart. Such happiness! There is a perfect timing when each piece of the puzzle is made to fit in, providing us with a clear view of the larger picture forming.

Several years ago I had stopped at the Jwalamukhi temple, and sat outside in the car, for some reason, hesitating to enter. And here was I now with time having passed by and Ma calling me directly into her bosom. There is no explanation for the pieces falling into place in this puzzle of my life.

The temple of Jwalamukhi is dedicated to the manifestation of the goddess in the form of fire. A blue flame, fed by natural gas, springs forth from the rock in the sanctum sanctorum, through which Goddess Jwalamukhi manifests herself. The famous temple with its dome-style architecture is revered as one of the 51 seats of the *Shakti peethas*.

When Akbar, the great Moghul Emperor, in the process of consolidating his empire, chanced upon the temple, he was taken aback by the phenomenon of the shooting flame and, on a later visit to the temple with his Empress Jodha Bai, as an offering to the goddess had the entire dome gilded with gold leaf.

I could sense an experience coming my way; my heart began to beat faster, a gentle quiver entered into my body and a nervousness came into my quickened step. I walked with my offering to the centre where the *jwala*, the fire beams from nowhere, bowing down to take her blessings, running my hand over the *agni* and moving with my *rudraksha mala* and little pendulum through the flames. The priest took the red vermillion powder from my hand and much to my surprise, opened the box and placed it right into the flame. With trembling hands I accepted my *prasada* and walked away. Something was awaiting me; I could sense it and was more curious than ever.

I had isolated myself from my other friends, at times like this wanting to be alone, away from the mundane chatterings of us mortals. A tall priest came up to me and guided me into a hall at the far end of the temple. There was a bed placed in the middle and beside it lay a towel, some water and other simple toiletries. The priest explained to me how every night the Mother Goddess would come and rest in this place so lovingly prepared for her. Every dawn the sheets were gently left unsettled, the water poured out, and the towel left damp from Ma's touch, showing that she had been there at a physical level. Today, I believe this story, but several years ago I would have laughed it away as a fable.

Stepping in to check out what it was all about, my gaze fell on a huge painting of Ma Kali! This was her; the same gentle, pretty nubile face, in deep hues of blue, tongue protruding, just as she had appeared to me. She did exist in this beautiful form as well, not just in the *rudra*, terrifying, form that everyone speaks and writes about! Her entire form was one of perfection and power. I could sense the *prana*, the life-force flowing through her. The long, black cascading stresses reminded me of the intensity of the *Kala ratri*, the dark night.

I wanted to take a picture of her beautiful form to place in my sacred space, a gentle reminder of the way she had appeared to me. The priest realised my intensity and allowed me to discreetly take a photograph and that I must say here, Ma Kali allowed me the privilege! For, in Chamba during my visit to the temple of Lakshmi Narayana, Ma Kali wouldn't allow me to take her picture.

The valley of Chamba reverberates with the vibrations of ancient temples, dating back to the 10th century. The six richly-carved temples lie in a row in the vicinity of the palace, three dedicated to Lord Vishnu and three to Shiva-Shakti. The Vishnu temples were built with two superimposed parasols with *shikhars* or spires and enshrined in their fold is the exquisite bronze image of *Chaturmurti*, Vishnu with four arms, remarkable for its naturalistic modelling. I seemed to be mesmerised by the wonder of it all and began taking pictures of the frescoes on the outer walls of the temples, capturing the tremulous longing and still exuberance set in stone.

The image of Ma Kali drew me to her and I felt amazing vibrations. A devotee had placed a red hibiscus flower at her feet; the flower that is most precious to her. I set my camera on her presence and focused animatedly, but the camera wouldn't click. I adjusted the range of focus, even distanced myself. It just wouldn't click. I walked over to the other fresco and tried out my camera. Click! Click! So I quickened my pace back to her. No! No! I bowed to Ma in reverence. Though I must explain, I never take pictures inside temples.

Arati at Kalibari

'Om klim kalikayei namaha.'
(Salutations! I attract she who is dark and powerful.)

In the midst of New Delhi, a stone's throw from the Gole Dakkhana, the post-office, bordering a forest patch is the Kali Mandir, a temple alive with Ma's reverberations. The Earth resounds with her might during the Friday evening *arati*. In all her silken and jewelled splendor, cutting a dark, formidable, enigmatic form, her deep, dark eyes smouldering the kinders of the *sadhaka's* soul, her tongue, the colour red of life's blood, hanging out, thirsting for annihilation of man's ego, waiting to be severed by the *khanda*, or head chopper, she carries in her hand.

To most people, Ma appears to be terrifying in form, yet for the evolving *sadhaka* she places herself in the heart *chakra*. This truly is her abode, the heart *chakra* of the subtle body, the throne of the air element, energising the physical heart, which circulates the life-force, and the blood, which carries it. *Rakta Kali*, the blood form of Kali, regulates the very beat and pulse of the human heart. Her benefic form, *Bhadra Kali* resides in the spiritual heart centre, which is located slightly to the right side of the chest, from which she gently directs our higher transformation, taking us to heights of self-realisation when we surrender to her. Is this not enough to truly understand her innate nature? As our mother, she will always be loving and consoling.

Dressed in the colour of passion, I ascended the flight of stairs to make an offering to Ma Kali, a little too early for the *arati*. Ma enjoys her celebration when darkness envelops the rest of us. The Earth below was sending gentle tremors into my being, making me seek refuge against a pillar, watching the last of the Sun's rays romancing the forest shadows. Drawing me into a deeper reverie were my powerful Kali *beeja mantras*; the surrounding vibrations were magical.

The rising crescendo beat of the *dhak*, the large drums, the hearkening bellow of the horns, and the clashing sound of metal from the *kashor ghanta*, the metal plate held by a rope pulled through and struck with a wooden stick, couldn't have provided a more powerful heralding of Maha Kali. The priest had a hypnotic sway to his bodily movements, invoking her with the *arati*, seemingly brought under her spell. The deep call emanating from the blowing of the conch shell commanded attention from every breath of my *prana*, my ego-less self, for the moment, bringing me to my knees with folded hands, reducing me to 'nothingness'.

The tolling of the temple bells and the sprinkle of *jal*, the blessing with water, brought me back into the present moment. The strains of Pandit Chhannulal Mishra of the Kirana *gharana*, a Benaras *gayaki*'s rendition of '*Dayo karo Maharani*', 'Have mercy O, queen of the goddesses!' ringing in my heart!

At midnight of the *Ashtami*, the eighth day of the Navaratri, I made my oblations to Ma with my *homa*, the fire ritual. I made an offering of the nudity of my body, mind and soul, enticing her with the sweet fragrance of sandalwood, *tagara*, *kasthuri*, *agaru*, *ashwagandha*, saffron and red roses. The flames arose to great heights, displaying their passion, a befitting tribute to her fiery nature. The play continued for over three hours, wishing away any sleep, sweeping me into its magical folds.

Ma made her presence known. She was always most benevolent with me. I would fall silent, no questioning, no seeking of answers; she knew what was best for me. The sound of temple bells would chime from nowhere, sensations would move through my entire being, lifting me into a wild crescendo of passion.

In *anjali mudra*, I rendered obeisance to Ma's form as Tripura Sundari.

'Aim hrim srim Om namas Tripurasundarya!'

(I bow to you, the most beautiful goddess of all waking, dreaming or sleeping worlds.)

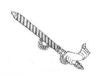

The Act of Sacrifice

'And if it is fear you would dispel, the seat of the fear
is in your heart and not in the hand of the feared.'
- Kahlil Gibran

I was 35 when I travelled to Chitkul, the last Indian village on the Indo-Tibetan border. They had recently opened up the area to visitors, and we must have been among the earliest groups to visit. Pristine purity, unspoiled, the landscape had retained its virginity. We walked across the clear glaciers, sighting a myriad of pink bramble bush roses.

One morning I strolled into the village, wanting to have a closer look at the simplicity of the people's humble existence. I stopped to watch the village belles stomping in huge cauldrons for the weekly wash, rinsing their clothes in the flowing stream, laying them out on huge boulders to take in the Sun and dry. Soon I found myself surrounded by elderly village women, the warmth of a hundred suns basking in deep etchings of aged lines of years gone by.

They stroked my hair and touched the nose-ring decorating my nose, held my hands, questioning me in a dialect of their native land, about the bangles on my wrist. They were curious to know the weight of the gold; surely, it has its play in every woman's heart. It was a bonding of womanhood, no matter where we hail from; the matters close to the heart are universal.

With dusk approaching, there appeared a hustle bustle of priests and laymen carrying a palanquin, decorated in colourful splendour. To me it seemed a wedding procession with the bride and her belongings, a majestic black goat in tow. The villagers told me that over the past few years they had fallen into bad luck, with no rain, no yield of crops and several unexpected deaths.

This was the local *devi*, the goddess, that they were carrying from her temple. It was a truly rare occasion, as she hadn't been moved for some 35 odd years. They were prepared to offer a sacrifice to appease her. I wanted to make my way out of the procession, but they wouldn't let me go.

The *bali*, sacrifice, to honour the goddess was being readied ceremoniously. I stood rooted to the Earth and watched the magnificence of a clean, swift, single drive of the revered sword remove the beautiful black goat from its head. What a display of passion in the form of deep red blood filling the night sky. I thought I was going to swoon; closing my eyes, I prayed that I would never be brought to perform such a sacrifice.

Escorted back to my tent, shutting myself away, I gave vent to a flood of tears renting the anguish and pain of a life being offered away. I hoped that the goddess would welcome the gentle creature offered to her.

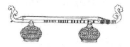

Nagakanya, Goddess of the Three Realms

'I bow to the Great Feminine, who abides in all beings
in the form of delusion.'
— Devi Mahatmyam

In *The Thousand Names of Bhavani*, Pandit Janakinath Kaul explains the *nagakanya* as one who became a serpent virgin to please Shambhu, Lord Siva, who loves serpents. "Becoming Shiva himself, one should worship Shiva," is a scriptural injunction. So becoming the beloved, the lover enjoys union with Him. Parvati, rapt in love for Shiva, assumed the charming form of *nagakanya* to gain His love. A serpent is also an emblem of the purity of love. In *Tantric* Buddhism, the *nagakanya* is the 'goddess of the three realms', she being an intermediary figure, and one who has special powers in air and water and can save us in difficulties.

The serpent symbol is very much in evidence in ancient Egypt and in the Mayan civilisation. The Mayan hierarchy of priests knew the secret of the serpent power, which was the basis of their magical and priestly arts. Almost every Mayan structure at Chichen Itza is adorned with serpent heads or motifs in some form.

Earlier I had dreams of serpents, but my first mystical experience with *Nagadeva*, the Serpent-lord, came to me in the valley of Jageshwar. The four-kilometre stretch of road through the valley quite enslaves the mind with its stupendous depths of *deodars* and blue pines. Their dense and heavy aroma seems to permeate the air. This is the site where Shiva's Maha Mritunjaya temple, dated back to the 13th century AD and first built by Raja Vikramaditya, nestles in the lap of Nature.

The Maha Mritunjaya *mantra* had been dwelling in my heart for over a year, always remaining on my lips when other words were unspoken. Its deep meaning resonated for me. "We worship the three-eyed Lord Shiva who nourishes and spreads fragrance in our lives. May He free us from the shackles of sorrow, change and death, effortlessly, like the fall of a ripe cucumber from its stem." My being could sense the astounding reverberations of the mystic surroundings.

I could barely wait to embrace the vibrations of the temple. My hand instinctively raised itself to strike the massive iron bell, an ancient accumulation of vibrations sent forth resounding waves through the blue pines, announcing yet another *sadhaka*. With devotional energies in abundance, paying my obeisance to Shiva as the three-eyed one, I bowed to him with deep reverence.

It was cold at three in the morning, the winds whispering through gaping crevices in the room, when I bathed my body, scented and oiled it with the thought of my Lord. Darkness prevailed as I stepped into the crisp air and walked down to the temple. The head priest guided me to sit by his side for the morning prayers. Coiled around the *Shivalingam*, raising its potent hood and deifying Shiva was a *naga*, a cobra, intricately depicting its magnificent markings in silver. I was allured into its hypnotic fold. The sharp crowing of a raven brought me back to the consciousness of the new morning. Stepping out, the wistfulness of Nature gently took me into her embrace.

'Sarvendriyagunabhasam.'— *Siva sutra 3.15*
(Who but Shiva can perceive the sense objects?)

The one who experiences the external waking world, the world of dreams, and the total oblivion of deep sleep is the Supreme Lord of *turiya*. Both the looker and the seen are the same supreme consciousness. The relationship of the senses and the sense objects is experienced while the senses perceive, delight in, and act on their respective objects. Shiva is the experience and Shiva is what is experienced. *Turiya* is a most beautiful Sanskrit word encompassing the power of consciousness to unify the waking, the dreaming and the sleeping states of a yogi.

Dusk brought with it the blessings of Shiva as the last rays of the Sun set upon the blue tree-line, casting shadows on the temples. It was time for the evening *maha abhishek*. I lost myself in the dim recesses of the temple in meditation and *mantra japa*, to be wakened by the Maharajji, the head priest, preparing for the *abhishek*. He placed the sacred mixture of yogurt, honey and turmeric in my hands and beckoned me to bathe the *Shivalinga* along with him.

In a reverie of worship my whole being was allured to the vibrations of the dark stone *Shivalinga*, when my middle finger, the finger of Saturn, seemed to trace the outline of the third eye engraved in it. This is the truly unique feature of this *lingam* at the Triyambakam temple. A tremulous ecstasy overcame me.

Laying back in bed, taking in the silence of a still night, in a deep contemplative mood of two days spent in close proximity with the cosmic powers, a chill seemed to crawl up my spine. Maybe I was beginning to sense something, straining my ears, only to pick up the whisper of the wind bellowing the secrets of the ancient sages through the *deodars*, rustling the needles of the blue pines.

I heard a heavy leaning against the wire mesh of my window and a hollow thumping of the hooded *naga*, serpent. Apprehension overtook my being, for when the time is not right, the conscious mind tends to intervene and block out an experience. I shut my eyes to this celestial visitor and began to shake my sister, who was lying beside me, for reassurance. She awoke and the *nagadeva* went into oblivion.

On the fifth day of the bright half of *Shravan*, Nag Panchami is celebrated all over India. Living cobras are venerated and fed sweetened milk, usually by women. People visit temples specially dedicated to snakes and worship them, Shiva temples being revered most highly. In the south of India, people craft images of the serpent from cowdung

229   *Nagakanya, Goddess of the Three Realms*

and place them on either side of the entrance of their homes in order to welcome the snake-gods and goddesses. The anthills are worshipped with pouring of milk over them.

The five-hooded *seshnaga* is made from mixing a fragrant pigment, turmeric, sandalwood and saffron, placed on metal plates and worshipped. The snake-charmers indulge in cobra–feeding as well. The experience at the Mandore fair in Jodhpur, attended by over a lakh people, where the region's snake-charmers bring their cobras to be worshipped, is captivating, the sway of the serpents literally leading one into a state of hypnosis.

At the edge of the backwaters, in the obscure town of Mannarsala near the capital Alleppey, is the auspicious place of the snake-king and queen, *Nagaraja* and *Sarpayakshi* presiding over a dense grove, in which thousands of idols of snakes are consecrated. Live serpents are found as well, though in less impressive numbers. Most *pambamkavus* or snake-groves have gradually vanished, but the king and queen are still worshipped at the temple run by a high-caste priestess.

Mevlana, My Beloved Master

'And if this day is not a fulfilment of your needs and my love,
then let it be a promise till another day.'
– Kahlil Gibran

Shiva is known as *Naganath*, the Lord of Serpents. The serpent represents the coiled energy of *kundalini*, the power that enables seeds to germinate and animals to procreate. Shiva, as Lord of all Vegetation created through his meditation and *tapas*, came to be known as *Vrikshanath*, the Lord of Trees. As the Lord of Beasts or wild animals, he is known as *Pashupati*. Shiva is the primordial *shaman* always in touch with Nature's mysteries. The ancient Cherokees and the Pueblo Indians also based their traditions on 'Nature worship', revering the Lord of Snakes, plants and animals.

During my earlier *sadhana*, I would experience a beautiful union of the male and female, black *naga* and *nagin*, which conjoined in perfect unison, moving up in great rhythm from my feet to my head. This continued over a period of several days. These experiences in my visions never created any fear; I began to understand their deeper meaning in reference to the awakening of the *kundalini shakti*.

Another time a beautiful brown *naga*, seemingly curious about me, moved around my bed, crawling up to my left, eventually raising his head in full-hooded grandeur to the left side of my face, looking over me whilst I lay in deep slumber.

Three weeks after an intense *sadhana*, during the alignment of the Earth, Sun and Saturn, I had the most amazing experience of a dark brown *naga* slowly coming up my body to reach my head. He spread his magnificent hood, opening his mouth wide and exposing his powerful fangs and the pink lining of his mouth. His flashing black eyes stared me in the eyes and he began to strike me at my forehead.

The awareness was so distinct and I was amazed at my state of calm, totally unafraid. With my right arm, I moved him away from my face and he stung me on the finger of my right hand and slithered off. The next day I rang up Ashokji, seeking guidance from him. He blessed me with a powerful *mantra*.

Mevlana was my beloved master, whose very manifestation I was seeking and deeply searching for in an earthly form! My search seemed to find its reflections in the thoughts and writings of this man I deeply revered, pouring my inner experiences into his fold, understanding the subtle nuances of the language he used in order to convey his subtle messages. He had the wisdom of the ancient sages. My life became enriched with experiences through his guidance and we traversed a deeper sacred space in many ways.

The deeper explanations to my experiences came through the guidance of this beautiful master: "You have the power of the *nagas* — earthly, atmospheric and heavenly. Astrologically you are a *naga kanya*, a serpent maiden, who moves like water, arising from the currents in the sea. *Nagakanyas* are a form of lightning, reverberating in the clouds and in space.

"Yet *nagas* are also mountains, so *nagakanya* is Parvati, Shiva's wife. And *nagas* are manifestations of elephants, so the *nagakanya* is also Matangi, the goddess who has the wild energy of the elephant. The northeast region of India and Guwahati in particular is famous for *nagakanyas*, who are the river-females. One of these, Ulupi, was the second wife of Arjuna (after Draupadi). Perhaps that is why you were born there. Above all, the *naga kanya* is the *yogini*. It is the *kundalini shakti* when its energy flows freely."

'Jai Gurudeva!'

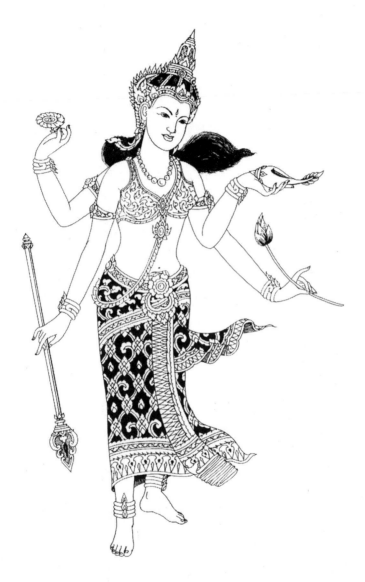

Jai Ma Guru

Nature is a Continuous Worship

'Om vishwa rupayaii namaha.'
(Salutations to she who is the form of the entire Universe.)

My whole existence became a temple, and Nature a continuous worship, the floating clouds a prayer, the ripples in the water transcendence and the mighty mountains a meditation! All I did was begin to be aware of my surroundings and tap into the vibrations of Mother Earth!

For me spirituality was never an exercise in being serious. Love, nurturing, prayer and laughter are the most sacred phenomena. I learned to reach out to the goddess and allowed her to take me into her fold, opening my heart and connecting to Nature's wonders through her. And she led me into the deep recesses of my soul. Ma became my guru in most ways.

Jai Ma Guru! The Mother Goddess guided me, sometimes working her ways through my revered earthly gurus who guided me to the path. Though my passion was clearly oriented towards Shiva, when the time was right, He led me to his consorts, to teach me the finer aspects of *sadhana*. They gently directed my thought process to certain disciplines necessary for *sadhana*, enlightening me through experiences with the *jnana*, knowledge of the *dasha mahavidyas*, the 10 great paths of knowledge.

In *Tantra Shastra*, the Supreme is worshipped and adored as the great primordial goddess, who manifests through 10 outstanding personalities or formations of wisdom. In the act of creation, the Supreme Mother opens herself to infinite space, creating the 10 directions of east, west, north, south, north-east, north-west, south-east, south-west, above and below. We experience life in 10 different ways through our 10 senses (*indriyas*, sense and motor organs) of skin, eyes, nose, ears, tongue, mouth, feet, hands, anus and genitals.

All the 10 *vidyas* lead one to the same ultimate reality. Yet each *vidya* is distinct from the other, each bestowing a particular cosmic function and special realisation of the one Supreme Reality. The great mystery and might of Kali, the power of deliverance and sound-force of Tara, the benign beauty and bliss of Sundari, the vast vision and space of Bhuvaneshvari, the Divine wrath and effulgence of Bhairavi, the lightning force of Chhinnamasta, the grandmotherly spirit and silent inertness of Dhumavati, the hypnotic and paralysing power of Bagalamukhi, the Divine joy and music of Matangi and the Lotus Goddess of Delight, Kamala.

One's inner aptitude and receptivity lead to the path of a particular goddess, to realise her inner might and strength and identify with her form. Choosing the path, we take to worshipping with adoration that particular aspect of the Divine, leading us on eventually to the next.

True mysticism or the deepest level of spirituality is concerned with personal transformation, directly experiencing God and becoming one with the Supreme Power, gradually ascending from the individual soul or *jivatma* to the Absolute. The goddesses guide us in this process, providing both the wisdom and the energy to bring it about, becoming themselves a visionary form of both the path and the goal, all at once. The goddess is the *yogini* and the power of yoga through which yoga fulfils itself like a mystic dance.

Prarabdha Unfurls Our *Karma*

'Your thoughts and my words are waves from a sealed memory
that keeps records of our yesterdays.'
– Kahlil Gibran

Prarabdha unfolds the *karmas* that must be experienced in the present life. Yet we need not make ourselves hostage to these if they are negative. There is no stopping us on the spiritual path if the fire to walk the path is there within us, though it is not an easy walk. The test of time will be extremely rigorous. Only the *vira sadhaka*, the brave one, who is truly sincere and has the *shraddha*, firm conviction, will be able to face all this. So take heed of all your trials and tribulations. At the end you will be shown a rainbow quite as surely as I am traversing this path myself.

As Vamadeva Shastri made clear to me, "The message of *karma* is one of freedom but a freedom that also has a responsibility along with it. The freedom of the artist to create is not a guarantee that what all artists create must be beautiful, nor does it allow the artist to neglect the rules and discipline of the art."

The freedom of *karma* is also bound to the field of natural law. This gives us a freedom of action but with consequences. (For example, you have the freedom to put your hand into a fire or not, but you don't have the freedom to put your hand into a fire and not get burned!)

Karma has been misunderstood from a responsible freedom of action into a kind of fate imposed upon us from the outside without our acceptance. But once we understand *karma*, then we see how we create our own destiny and direct our lives to a higher goal.

Karma only means that we are experiencing what we need for our soul's development. We are not bound to anything else in this life. It doesn't mean that we shouldn't love and share with others, trying to avoid bad *karma* at the cost of eliminating all contact or adventure. If we were meant to be alone all the time, we would not have hands that reach out, a mouth that expresses love, eyes that envisage beauty, and a body that unfolds into another's while making love. We would not be able to speak because there would be no reason for communication.

However, the only person that one has to rely on for a spiritual experience is oneself. And we can't gain this without grace and love; we weren't meant to. Certainly life is not a bed of roses. But that doesn't mean we can't get through it with grace, love and humour! So we must get rid of 'guilt', 'hellfire', 'damnation', 'mortal sin', and all other misconceptions that have kept people under control for centuries. True spirituality has to be positive and become a bastion for help, love, giving and sharing; not for avoidance of sin, bad *karma* or pain.

The word *karma* has been bantered around and misused so much that everyone has become confused. Too often it is misunderstood to be some tremendous backlash — some kind of wrath from the 'great beyond'. This misconception has made people almost as repressed as they are judgmental. It makes us fear-based rather than aspiration-based. Every emotion such as anger, vengeance, or hurt seems sure to carry with it a *karmic* barb, but this is not the reality.

In the original texts, the concept of *karma* had nothing to do with judgment. There is no God sitting above and passing judgments. How could He be, when he is omnipotent, holding and loving you? We must learn to stop using *karma* as a hammer over our own heads! One hears people say, "I can't leave my husband and the kids even though he beats me because it is my *karma*." Such a person may in actuality be *karmically* destined to 'grow' through the experience of pushing that abusive person out of her life! God did not mean for anyone to come down here to suffer endlessly.

We are all tiny particles moving with universal energies as in a huge duststorm. It is the cosmic order that links us as individuals together. People use *karma* as an excuse to cling to the familiar and not make efforts in life. You can't say that you live with someone awful or difficult, who doesn't understand your core, because it is your *karma*! You do not have to put up with an impossible kid, painful in-laws or an unsatisfying job, marriage, relationship, health or anything because it is one's ordained *karma*!

The one obligation that we do have *karmically* is to finish whatever we begin. So if you start a relationship — either a romance or a friendship — and you are the major instigator behind it, and somewhere along the line you outgrow the relationship, or it outgrows you, your *karmic* obligation, unfortunately, says that you must be the one to go in, face the relationship, and end it! This principle is the same with jobs or anything else we undertake.

Listen to your 'own soul' and its 'inner voice'. We are moving on from one millennium to another, and all around us people tell of the *karma* they've created in themselves and on this very Earth that keeps everything stuck in the mire. I don't think we should allow anyone to treat us as less than Divine! We all have a godliness existing within us! "*Aham Brahmasmi*" as Adi Shankaracharya preached in the *Shastras*, "I am Brahman". One needs to love and nurture oneself, only then can we learn to love and nurture another, and this is also part of our *karma*!

We are afraid of not being loved, but does it really matter? The most beautiful lesson I learned through my experiences in life was to be concerned with loving, just loving without any conditions or expectations. It is not quite so easy, but can unfold a wondrous state of mind. It takes away from any attachments or material expectations, or the need to control.

Man's greatest need is to feel needed, but when we experience that the whole existence needs us or else we would not have been born here, love will then blossom in our lives. When we trust that the whole Universe is on our side, then we need not fear *karma*. We cannot only make a better future, we can step outside of time altogether.

Love on the Run

'If this is my day of harvest, in what fields have I sowed the seeds,
and in what unremembered seasons?'
- Kahlil Gibran

M y son preferred the company of people beyond his age, being
less tolerant with children of his own age. He had grown up to
the harsh realities of the world, moving through the turbulence of his
parents' marital discord and his mother's deep insecurities. He tried
his best to play the role of an adult, but kept slipping somewhere, grop-
ing his way through the dark.

One was aware of the excitement about a young woman who had
eloped from college, seeking her happiness in the throes of romance.
Sometimes life is scripting another story, steering us away from the
throb of deeper love, bringing in its wake a surge of upheaval.

The urgency in my son's tone unnerved me; the tragedy of the hour
pierced my heart. The gentle couple, friends of my son, had met with a
terrible motorcycle accident, the scarf around her neck dragging her to
the ground, her unsheathed head mercilessly becoming a strike force
against cruel fate. The doctors in the emergency room couldn't seem to
revive her to consciousness and had given her up as dead.

My son rushed me to her bedside, his frightened eyes drawing all
my inner resources. They allowed me in to the ICU, my hand reaching

into the recesses of my handbag, frantically searching out my magic potion of the Mother Goddesses.

I touched her pulse point at the wrist and drew my inner guidance to seek the deeper answers to the quest of her life.

I emerged from her dark confines, hopeful in my faith of the *shakti*, force within, comforting her better half with my warm hold, "She is going to be with you." The doctors on attendance had no hope; the medical sciences through their powerful monitors seemed to have sealed her fate already. They made me nervous for a moment, and I decided to drive to my spiritual guide for support.

Past 11 in the night, we drove through his gates, much to his surprise. I drew out their picture in the presence of my son and seeked further guidance. "What do you want Shambhavi? Whatever you wish will be. You have already touched her somewhere; what did you apply?"

We were taken aback by his powerful intuition, and I asked my son to leave us to the confines of privacy. "No, let him be a witness to what his mother is doing." Turning to my son, "Since you have come with your mother, to create faith in you the Mother Goddess will work her magic."

He instructed me to return immediately to the hospital and place my hand on her forehead. I confided my fear of the unknown, unable to bring myself to touch her head, which was so hurt by the aggression of the impact. 'Go Shambhavi,' his silence dismissed our presence.

We drove to the hospital in a deathly silence, bonding deeply as mother and son. I had no words to comfort his questioning heart. "Ma what was Ashokji trying to say?" His childlike fear was answering my deep fears. I drew strength from the silence and began my conversation with the Mother Goddess.

We walked in at well past 1 a.m., no one seemed to stop me move through the realms of healing ways. Standing by her side, my soul reached out to her, and a deep prayer rose from my being, 'Ma, bless them with a happy life together.'

A flow of compassion swept through me, washing away any traces

Love on the Run

of human fear, my hand reaching out to reassure her with Ma's benevolence. She moved and my heart filled with joy.

Outside I held Kamal , her husband, close to my being, whispering into his ear, the strength for both of us to surrender to her will. My prayers found its voice and softly asked him to continuously keep the flow of love reaching out to his gentle beloved. I wanted him to believe in my belief. We were being strong for each other. His pained eyes were searching for the truth.

A new strength permeated my being, and I reassured my nervous son, that she would gain consciousness on Saturday and would win back her lost thoughts, no matter what the dictates of science had to say. My sacred space comforted me later that hour of dawn, sending me into the throes of a peaceful slumber.

The Saturday found an excited son exclaim over the phone, "Ma she recognised me, saying, 'Hi fatso'!" We rallied by the two of them, reassuring them of the blessings and abundance of the Universe.

'And when the shadow fades and is no more,
the light that lingers becomes a shadow to
another light.'

Brahma Unfolds in Stone

'Brahma, Lord of Creatures (*Prajapati*), all these forms that have
come into being are not different from you. Whatever wish we
offer, may that come true.'
— *Yajur Veda*

Brahma was resplendent in his divinity, in his serene calm! The three
heads seemed to be set in stone with a light sandstone colouring,
as He appeared to me at the early morning of half past six. I was a bit
confused by His appearance, for at that moment I perceived the
appearance to be of the Great Trinity — Brahma, Vishnu and
Maheshvara, but much later I became clear with the understanding
that it was surely my *darshan* of Brahma only.

The learned say that one should keep secret the Divine experiences
with which one is blessed, or else they stop happening, but I want to
share these experiences with all my fellow-*sadhakas* for the benefit of
all genuine seekers. And I must dare to say that even after sharing my
experiences they never stopped happening; on the contrary, they
increased manifold. My *sadhana* continued with the same zest and
passion, and before me unfolded other blessings in the form of the Ten
Mahavidya Goddesses and several other mystical experiences which I
continue to share.

Hari, as I preferred to call him, instead of Harry, was visiting me from New York; a man of quiet nature, very deep in his thoughts. My own long stays in New York were spent at his home. Every morning he'd silently step into my room to say his morning *gongyo*, the Buddhist chant in front of the *gohonzon*, before leaving for work. I guess the chanting would remain in my subconscious mind. He'd make me my morning tea, pat my head and leave for work. Several years later I took to chanting his *mantra* myself, once in awhile.

During his visit, Hari and I drove down to Jaipur to view some traditional Indian silver jewellery. What a riot the pink city of Jaipur is! History seems to tell its own story: the busy bylanes picturesque with the Rajasthanis in their colourful turbans and brilliant *ghagara-cholis*, the long skirts with backless tops, maidenly arms filled with bangles of varying hues, accompanied by the loud chatter of the local dialects. It is simply mesmerising!

At four in the afternoon, the shopkeeper convinced us to drive to Ajmer and Pushkar, though none of this was in our schedule. We drove through the desert landscape following the setting Sun and winding through the low hills under a moonlit sky, we reached Ajmer Sharif round 10 in the night. The place seemed quite peaceful, not madly abuzz with people. I am quite shy of crowds, and never appreciated being touched by people, so most times I avoid busy places.

The *dargah* has its own magic, reverberating with the blessings of Babaji, the deep aroma of the red roses, incense wafting through the air, the prayer of hope on every person's lips, the flash of ardour in every pair of eyes seeking Allah. Amidst this mystical atmosphere, I wanted to drop to my knees with hands folded with the expression of '*Masha Allah*', by the Grace of Allah!

I chose a beautiful green satin *chaddar*, the shawl worked into its edges with brilliant gold braid and tasselled on all sides, placed the incense, *itar*, the perfume, red roses and *tabarruk*, the sweet offerings. My being was feeling the stimulation of the surroundings and stepping into the *dargah*, there was a tranquillity filling my inner space. With reverence I placed the *chaddar* and offerings in the Pir Saab's hands and silently awaited an acknowledgement, experiencing a complete blankness in my mind.

He held the *chaddar* over my head and suddenly I experienced a heavy, large hand weighing my head down, sharpening my state of awareness. I looked up bewildered at who was placing a hand on my head. The green colour seemed to scintillate a green aura of the light shining through, and there was no hand; the Pir Saab's hands were firmly holding the *chaddar* on both sides.

Ajmer Sharif Dargah is famous for its ability to fulfil our wishes. Most people go there with a wish in their hearts and they say when the wish is fulfilled, one must return in gratitude. Somehow no wish arose in my heart at that special moment, not that there weren't any wishes to be fulfilled. There are many from invoking the Mother Goddess to experiencing the hues of love expressed in my life. A myriad of red threads are seen tied in knots, each encasing a wish to come true.

The night was beautiful and I was happy sitting back in the car, cherishing the Universe. Moreover I was on my way to seek fulfilment in the eventual Trinity!

It was nearing the midnight hour when we reached Pushkar, the abode of Lord Brahma. A veritable alluring desert night, reflections of a near full Moon sending deep ripples across the magical waters of the Pushkar lake.

It was impossible to contain one's self from the pull of the waters, and I found myself running down the steps, slipping my hands into the coolness of the water, filling my palms, making an offering into space. My visit to the Brahma temple seemed to make me come full circle, for now I had paid obeisance to the Trinity — Brahma, Vishnu and Maheshvara.

In *Tantra*, Brahma is the embodiment of the creative power, ruling over destiny, making it imperative to the *sadhaka* to become one with Brahma. Through the power of identification, the power of creativity can work in an individual at all levels. Saraswati, the feminine energy or consort of Brahma is the *shakti*, the creative power, without which no act of creation can manifest. Brahma and Saraswati are the inseparable 'creative aspect' and 'creative energy', forming the cosmic couple.

This dualism is present in every worldly relationship and the unity of these two principles has great significance in the path of *Tantric* love. When both partners work on expressing their higher ideals, all aspects of their intimate relationship manifest an inner spiritual significance and the identity of Brahma and Saraswati.

Ma Lakshmi Leads Me to her Consort

'We adore Lakshmi, who has the nature of supreme peace
and the luster of pure gold,
whose form is radiant, wearing gold and possessing all ornaments.
who caries a golden chalice and a golden lotus, whose hands
give gold, the original power,
the Mother of all, who dwells at the side of Lord Vishnu.'
– *Lakshmi Dhyanam*

In its role as preserver of the cosmic order, the Divine is called Vishnu. His is the force that maintains all existence and keeps everything in harmony. Ashokji, my gentle spiritual teacher, had given me a Vishnu *mantra* to chant over the months, asking me to pay obeisance to Lord Vishnu and seek his blessings at Badrinath.

I took the offbeat route to Badrinath, driving through the *bugyals*, the meadows of Chopta, lush green, a mass with zillions of wild flowers. The tinkling bells around the flock of sheep seemed to be the only sound. The night sky heralded a twinkling of stars so bright that one almost felt we could reach out and handpick them. Such are the blessings from the cosmic pulse of Nature. These were truly ethereal moments, freeing my soul from earthly *bandhans*, human ties.

The long stretch of drive through the dark, dense forests still carried the vibrations of Lord Rama on his way to *banavas* (exile). The intense throb from the deep meditations of *rishis* and seers from ancient times reverberated in the background. In my joyous exuberance, I would halt the car, alight and run like a child through the forests, every pulse in my body accepting the grace of divinity's mark throughout the ages. Nature brought out the wildest and the purest emotions in me, throwing every caution to the winds of heaven.

The gates at Joshimath shut at 4 p.m. because driving at night through these roads is not considered at all safe. The drive proved to be arduous and unsafe owing to the heavy spate of the River Alakhananda flowing through the valley. I reached at half past seven, and for some unseen reason was just going to continue to drive through the gates for my *darshan* at dawn. It was like a calling; there was no stopping me. Strangely, no one had closed the gates, which were still partially open.

I instructed Sanjay, who faithfully drove me to my abode of blessings, not to stop and to continue driving right through, fearlessly. He was nervous as the police heavily man most of the posts. I placed my hand on his shoulder and he just drove through the gates. No one around looked our way; unbelievable are the mystical ways of the Universe when your call has come!

A kilometre down the road, he pulled the car over in sheer nervousness, "Madam, have you no fear of anything?" I was bold, travelling on my own. I drew strength from my fervent prayers. The night grew dark, with the Moon playing hide and seek behind the magnanimous mountain peaks. We were driving through a gorge. The only light showing us the way was the beam of the car. The road was giving way in several places with the heavy flow from overhead waterfalls at times swaying the car through the force of its torrid currents. The Alakhananda appeared trapped, at times turbulent, crashing down its boulder-strewn riverbed.

The night had an eerie silence about it, with only ethereal souls inhabiting the surroundings. I could sense a fear arising in Sanjay, as he gently reminded me it was a mistake to drive through the night. My heart was soaring, a passionate fervour gripping my being. I wanted to romance the unknown, the dark night, and experience the wild rush of the waters sounding like a million waterfalls rushing down to the Earth. I burst out into Divine song, chanting my powerful *mantras*, and Sanjay joined my reverie, drowning out the tempestuous ardour of the river.

It was a surreal night. We arrived at a fork in the road and had no clue which direction to proceed in. I was prepared to take a chance, when to my left, outside my window, a magnificent, great Himalayan owl stared me in the face, mesmerising me with its awesome magical wonder. Spreading its wings to its full grandeur, it arose, swooped in front of the windshield and turned right!

I received my directions, and turning right followed the great bird's flight, with a deep sense of nearness to Lord Vishnu overcoming me. The owl is the *vahana*, vehicle for Ma Lakshmi, who has the nature of supreme peace and the lustre of gold, whose form is radiant, carrying a golden chalice and a golden lotus, whose hands bestow showers of gold, who is the original power, the mother of all, dwelling at the side of Lord Vishnu. Lakshmi rises out of the lotus from the cosmic ocean. She is the Goddess of Wealth, beauty, fertility, love and devotion, like the Greek Aphrodite and the Roman Venus.

We left the rush of the river behind and began a gradual climb, reaching Vishnu's abode much past the midnight hour. Making my way through the impregnable silence of the night, I knocked on a door emitting strains of a faint light. A priest emerged, rather taken aback at seeing me and I asked to be taken to the head priest. We made our way through an alley and entered a narrow corridor. We were offered large cushions to seat ourselves on, while a lot of whispered conversations were taking place behind closed doors.

The doors opened and a beautiful man emerged, youthful virility in his aura, a strength of unknown sages, and a vermillion red shawl wrapping his shoulders. Golden thread work matched on the cap and the shawl. I was taken aback with his grandeur. He questioned me, expressing much surprise at the timing of my visit, suggesting how dangerous travel can be during a dark night in these high mountain regions. I lowered my eyes in reverence and softly said it was the calling of Lord Vishnu; no other reasoning was necessary.

　　　　　　　　　　　　　　　Ma Lakshmi Leads Me to her Consort

They ushered me to a suite nearby, overlooking the Alakhananda, and slipping into the warmth of the soft quilts, saying my little, 'thank you' to my Lord, I drifted into a deep slumber. Within a few short hours, I was woken up for the morning *Maha Abhishekam*. Hot water from the spring was carried up to my room. Having bathed, stepping out I found it was still dark and a chill rented the air.

The temple has the *garbha griha*, where the deity is seated and the *mandapam* for pilgrims to assemble for darshana. The *Skanda Purana* describes how Adi Guru Shankaracharya, in pursuance of Divine orders, dived into the Narad *kund* and recovered the idol of Lord Vishnu, which he duly re-enshrined here in the 8th century AD.

The most intricately woven leaves of the holy *tulsi*, basil, are delicately put together with white flowers into long strands. Taking some garlands with me, I did a *parikrama* of the temple and was ushered inside. There were very few people, for luckily it was off-season. The Rawalji, as the head priest is referred to, stepped in with a lot of fanfare. Lining both sides were *pundits* readying for *puja*. Unlike other temples, at Badrinathji only the head priest worships the main deity.

The crescendo of the Vedic chanting along with the ardent chiming of bells sent reverberations through the temple walls. The Rawalji began the *maha abhishek puja*, removing all the elaborate decorations of Lord Vishnu. The idol of Lord Badrivaishal, as Vishnu is called here, is made of black stone. The Lord, seated in *padmasana* posture, is bathed and covered with a wrap of fresh *tulsi* leaves and tiny white flowers.

The fragrance of *tulsi* and other Himalayan herbs used in the offering, infused the crisp early morning air. The sheath of *tulsi* was removed from the idol and Rawalji, looking at me, aimed a large piece into my lap, incense wafting through the air. The fire *arati* brought with it tremendous high sounding vibrations through my being, filling my eyes with unshed tears as I held up my hands, holding the sacred *tulsi* in surrender. Leaving the temple, I had a deep feeling of being blessed, happy and divine.

Stepping into the sunshine, the early morning rays seem to romance the flowing waters of the Alakhananda, showering these blessings with a Divine joyousness. The skies wore a brilliance of sheer azure, bringing a prayer to my lips.

> 'And how shall you rise beyond your days and nights
> unless you break
> the chains which you at the dawn of your understanding
> have fastened around your noon hour. '
> - Kahlil Gibran

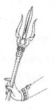

Miraculous Journey to Kedareshvara

'Shiva is the experiencer and the object of experience.
Shiva is the goal of *sadhana*.'

On one of my yearly journeys to Kedarnath, the Himalayan shrine dedicated to Shiva, I was truly blessed with Shiva's *darshan*. The Kedareshvara temple at Kedarnath, dedicated to Lord Shiva, houses the ninth of 12 *jyotirlingas*, the shafts of stone, symbolic of Shiva. The arduous climb to an elevation of 3,500 metres through waterfalls alongside the crystal clear water of the Mandakini river, opens up to an expanse of pasture land in a lush valley. Standing forth majestically is a 1,000-year old temple built in the 8th century by Adi Sankaracharya.

I was making this trip solely to pray for a dying friend. His liver had given way, his spleen wasn't functioning, and he knew he was dying — a beautiful yet deeply trying experience. He would call me long distance: "Ma, save me. I don't want to die, I want to live, Ma!" All of his 35 years seemed to be pleading to cling on to life. And I gave him my word that I would pray for his life, much against the will of my spiritual teacher who saw this as a heavy *karmic* case and advised me to stay away. But I have always loved a challenge and took it upon myself to invoke the Mother Goddess to save my friend.

By evening, I had arrived at Shiva's abode and prepared myself for the evening *arati*. I paid my respects to the Maharajji presiding over the *math*, sat with him for a while, and then stepped into the beautiful temple of Kedarnath. The inside walls are exquisitely embellished with mythological figures. The vibrations there reverberated with Shiva. They made way for me to pass through, and I stood in the enclosure to one side, my soul soaring to the heights of bliss, for I was in the very presence of my Lord Shiva. Standing in front was an elderly *sadhaka* lost in a song to Shiva and I wondered at the purity of his *bhakti*, utter devotion. As if he read my mind, the elderly *sadhaka* turned around and we locked eyes, and I turned my gaze to the floor in reverence.

The *arati* at Kedarnath is like an experience from another world. The very walls scream out Shiva's name and the flames of the *arati* literally singe one's entire being — one is transported into a state of 'no mind'. Truly, I have experienced liberation through the fusion of transcendental or pure consciousness and spirit. At the end of the *arati*, I stood to one side, taking in the residues of the deep vibrations, when I noticed the elderly *sadhaka* walking towards me. He bowed down and touched my feet. I had no idea how to acknowledge his respectful act. I think I stepped back in surprise, and he walked past me into the cold autumn night.

That night I retired to my spartan room after a moonlit walk down the road, taking in the presence of Shiva with every breath, in admiration of the vastness and beauty of the valley. The night rendered me cold, with the chilly winds coming through the crevices of my windows, with no heating in the room. I wrapped myself in whatever possible and slid into the confines of my sleeping bag, dozing off to the lullabies of celestial beings.

Waking the next morning to the splendours of a beautiful day, the rays of the Sun were warming the temple walls. I climbed up the mountaintop to collect some water from the source of the clear mountain spring of *Dhudh Ganga*, literally the flow of milk from the Ganga. Waterfalls are forms of *shakti* carrying the goddess's energy, her spiritual and healing power that flows downward from the higher

Miraculous Journey to Kedareshvara

worlds. The waters of these springs contain healing and rejuvenating forces, bringing out the magical properties of the Earth. Amazingly, my spiritual teacher visualised this flow, though never having been there himself, had asked me to carry this water back for my friend's life. The water was flown to him. Though given no chance to live, he was revived and managed to live for another two-and-a-half years.

Seva and Maya

'Udyamo bhairavah.'
– Siva Sutra 1.5
(Effort is itself Bhairava.)

In the afternoon, Maharajji of the Kedarnath temple sent for me and asked me to go into the temple and perform *seva*, but I retorted that no way would they allow a woman into the temple at this hour, when they bathe and prepare the *Shivalingam* for the evening *arati*. But Maharajji sent me in with his escort. In my nervousness, I quickly picked up a broom and began sweeping, hoping no one would notice me and throw me out. Suddenly, the broom was taken out of my hands. I looked up to see the same elderly *sadhaka* from the evening before. I folded my hands in *pranaam*, and he led me to the powerful statue of Parvati Ma, Shiva's consort, which is over a 1,000-years old, and asked me to begin performing her *shringar*, adornment.

Awestruck, I stuttered that Maharajji had sent me to sweep the floor. In fluent English, he gently said, "This is your blessing that you are allowed to adorn the goddess. Since the Navaratri, the nine-day festival, no one has touched Ma. Everyday I request Maharajji to allow me this honour, and he invariably says, 'Not today'! Will you please grant me one wish? Allow me to pour just one mug of water over her." With his sheer humility, he humbled my entire being.

With trembling hands I removed Ma's *shringar*, bathed her gently with hot water, and adorned her in beautiful red silk and jewels. What ecstasy was experienced! My eyes were brimming with tears and my whole body was quivering. A young priest asked me, "Who are you? Are you a *sadhvi*?" Embarrassed, I had to tell him the truth — that I was no *sadhvi*; just an ordinary woman seeking her Shiva. The elderly *sadhaka* then beckoned me to my additional amazement to help bathe the *Shivalinga*.

My hands and my entire being trembled as I bathed the *lingam*. Even the boiling hot water wouldn't scorch my hands, and when I finished, my hands were red like the stains of red *alta*. Gradually I had grown numb. The experience seemed to be one of intense purification. A priest softly said, "You must be the only woman who has ever been allowed to enter the temple and bathe Ma and the *Shivalingam*. Consider yourself highly blessed." My eyes welled up with joy and as I stepped out into the sunshine, I wanted to leap into the skies and scream, 'Shiva! Shiva!'

My tryst with Shiva was not over yet. I decided to walk down from the temple that evening at 4 p.m., despite everyone asking me not to. I set out alone, and within the hour it was dark, though the moonlight above lit my path. I had no fear of the unknown until a young man stepped into my path and offered to escort me. After a couple of hours, we stopped to find a torch as it had become dark with clouds arising to obscure the light of the Moon.

A tall man stood before me, nearly blocking my path and said he'd protect me on my journey downhill. He insisted, "Sister, I will walk with you and look after you." He was reeking with alcohol, and I declined his offer explaining I wasn't alone and needed nobody, but he insisted. At that point, I wasn't afraid and continued on my climb downhill. He kept stepping over to my side and began to place his arm around my shoulder, saying "Sister, don't be afraid."

I was beginning to be afraid. The mind plays the strangest of games, and our conditioning that has taught us to mistrust the Universe and humanity plays havoc with our being. My patience began to run thin and I reprimanded him gently, but he continued to come over to me and place his hand on my shoulder. Panic gradually began to over-come me and I started chanting my *mantras* silently for protection, until the last straw came when he placed his hand at my lower back.

In a moment of sheer madness, losing all reasoning and control, I turned around and with my stick lashed out at him, pushing him to the ground. My guide lifted a huge rock to crush him and I managed to push it out of his hand, realising the *karmic* repercussions of taking a life. Duly shaken, after walking a few steps, I turned to look back. The man had disappeared; there was no one there!

In my deep consciousness I realised this Divine *lila*, and broke down and sobbed like a child. My guide was so taken aback, he put his arm around me and comforted me, "Don't worry, sister!" I froze, distressed with the sheer reality that after all, my mind took over and was play-ing games with me, blinding me from recognising and seeing the truth.

Who was that *man*? Why was *his* touch ever so gentle on my shoul-der, most certainly not the touch of a drunken man at all? Even his hand placed at my *muladhar chakra* was ever so gentle. Caught in the web of *maya*, I seem to know no better and see no clearer!

When I narrated the incident to my spiritual teacher, he said: "Close your eyes and tell me who did you see; whose touch did you really feel?" I knew the answer! All my *sadhana* is for the One Divinity, and yet I was unable to recognise him when he came to me. A lifetime's experience drowned in *maya!*

A *sadhaka's* path is abundantly interesting and yet there has been deep anguish, insecurity and impatience to know the larger picture. But the single most powerful factor has always been my deep seeking of the Divine. Never has anyone been able to distract my attention from my Lord Shiva, and this passion has shaped my life.

I am always subconsciously trying to surrender while consciously my mind finds ways of drawing me further into the web of *maya*. Yet my web is one of love, searching for that benign, all-consuming love, where one sees the partner to be the Lord's own presence.

I have learned that there is one great value in living life fully and making mistakes, for if you survive and learn from them, the learning comes from your own experience and the knowledge is reliable. I sat at my teacher's feet and questioned him deeply about love and he compassionately said to me, "Surrender, and I will promise you the offering of pure love, the love you search."

Whatever you desire will eventually come to you; this is the magnanimity of Nature and Mother Earth. For one living and experiencing *Tantra*, and more so for one striving to be an *aghori*, for *aghora* is simply a path of intense devotion to the great Mother Goddess Kundalini — the entire world is Her temple and playground. All that happens to us is not 'ordinary' or 'coincidental'. I believe we must treat every event as a message from the great mystery, which makes us realise that life is a Divine *lila*, the play of God. One truth was very clear to me – nothing happens without her *anugraha*, her Divine grace.

Divinity Beyond All Norms

'Even as he ascends to your height and caresses
your tenderest branches that quiver in the Sun,
so shall he descend to your roots and shake them in their
clinging to the Earth.'
— Kahlil Gibran

My experiences have shown me that the Divine is beyond all religions and religious practices. At one point of my *sadhana*, I would chant powerful *mantras* to the background music of Sufi saints; the louder the music the more passionate my encounter with trance. My wonderful older son, Nikhil Arjun, who patiently saw me through this phase, would ask me, "Ma, how can you concentrate on a *mantra* while listening to Sufi music? They don't go together."

I must mention here for the benefit of other *sadhakas* that the path of *siddha yoga* is one in which the guru usually awakens the disciple's inner *shakti*, the *kundalini*, through the yogic process of *shaktipat*. As a result the seeker undergoes various spiritual experiences. But *shaktipat* or *kundalini* awakening can occur even without the guru, as explained by Swami Muktananda of Ganeshpuri.

The *kundalini* can become activated through austerities, *mantra yoga*, intense devotion, by the guru's grace received in a previous life, or as a result of *sadhana* in a previous life. Sometimes one receives initiations from a saint or deity in a dream or through visionary experiences like an overwhelming urge to isolate oneself from the world, burning sensations in the body, seeing snakes, tigers or fire. Yet due to ignorance, one doesn't realise it is the awakening of the *kundalini*, nor does one know how to utilise these experiences to reach the Divine goal.

We make our own roads, each one of us, and whether we travel freely and joyously or lonely, miserable and burdened by illnesses and anger, it is entirely up to us. When we gain access to a psychic or spiritually formative energy, we begin to enjoy a strong sense of well-being and transcendence. Even if the path happens to be non-existent, with the power of positive thinking we can ensure that the path is formed as and when we walk it.

Trials, pain and heartache visit all of us now and then. We must keep the balance within, for these too shall pass. The motionless centre around which all movements take place is 'you'. Cherish, love and nourish this inner 'you', for the only 'constant' in our lives is change! We must all learn to channel our life force and spiritual energies, starting from this very moment.

Simplicity of Spiritual Fervour

'Verily you are suspended like scales between your sorrow and your joy.
Only when you are empty are you at standstill and balanced.'
— Kahlil Gibran

E ach one of us is born and one day each will die. Between these two extraordinary events is the mysterious process that we call 'life'. Life is a precious gift for each one of us. Yet it is very easy to get so caught up in the daily chores necessary to maintain our existence that we go about our business as if life were nothing special at all! Divinity, however, reminds us rather gently that life is something special! Life is a wonderful adventure and an inner quest for something sacred! It is a great enigma to be solved.

Through my experiences I learned to unravel this enigma and make it a celebration, despite the pain and problems that I kept stumbling upon. Entering into the spiritual world, I began awakening to my inner self and the journey began leading me through utter confusion to deep inner meaning, from fear to faith, from feeling alone at times in a hostile surrounding to be at one with everything, and from ennui (world-weariness) to a life filled with magic. In short, I learned to brave the winds!

All too often we unquestioningly accept the norms of our culture and simply live the lives that others expect of us. Realised masters urge us not to follow the herd unconsciously, but to search for our own answers. We are all born *alone*, we will die *alone* and in between we each have an individual responsibility for our own development.

We can either bumble along in the semi-conscious state that we think of as normal or we can wake up to the miracles of a beautiful existence! We can either mindlessly accept what we have been told or else transform our lives into a journey of 'personal discovery'!

I chose the path of personal discovery, discovering in its wake that *nothing is permanent* — this body, this moment of time, these emotions — all are impermanent. Yet the beauty of life never ceases to exist, even in this impermanence. Looking deeply into a lotus flower, I could perceive its impermanent nature quite clearly, at the same time, still enjoy its fragile beauty and value its preciousness.

In my silent sojourns into the deep Himalayan mountains, whether looking at the early rising Sun, counting the seven colours of the rainbow, stepping gently on the morning dew on blades of green grass, admiring the stoic silence of ripened wheat fields or catching glimpses of a shooting star from a night sky, I began to enjoy each 'special moment' with a quiet prayer. Seeing deeply the impermanent nature of these beautiful experiences, their transformation and sudden disappearance, they taught me not to despair, but only to more carefully attend to these little miracles of everyday life. I felt like a child taking its first steps in ease and freedom, moving through the door of the present moment to realms beyond time and space.

The Temple of the Body

'Sariram havih.'
- Siva Sutra 2.8
(The body is the offering.)

A yogi who has offered his body to the fire of awareness, wherever he may be — in heaven or in our mortal world — considers everything to be in the nature of consciousness only. He submits all distinctions, *karmas*, sins and sorrows to the purifying fire of yoga and becomes one with Shiva, the Supreme.

Through myths, symbols and rituals of the timeless goddess, we can unravel and understand who we once were in order to appreciate who we are now at this particular time and place. And whether we see the goddess as creator, destroyer, mother, priestess or seductress, we can discover her many personalities in ourselves and learn to identify with each one of them as our own expression.

A balanced nurturing of body, mind and soul is required for the full blossoming of our true well-being. The body is our temple and must be revered in every way. *Tantra* trains us to believe that our body is a living miracle, a beautiful gift from the higher powers of the Universe. We must learn to protect, love and cherish this human body, and it will reveal great mysteries to us. Indeed in *Tantra*, the entire Universe is said to dwell in our own bodies, which is a God's way of manifesting in His own creation.

Often we are critical about our bodies, forming dislikes for our pot-bellies, small breasts, heavy thighs, balding hairline, or whatever it may be, and giving vent to these physical limitations with negative statements, like 'No one will accept me', 'I am too fat', 'I want to be all muscle and strong,' and so on. These thoughts usually manifest in our lives when there has been a lack of love or of a nurturing relationship either in our adult lives or as children.

Through spirituality we can heal our psyche and learn to accept and be gentle with ourselves. We need to look into our eyes in the mirror and say to ourselves, 'I love myself just the way I am!' We must learn to speak to our bodies and listen carefully to what they are saying through headaches, tension, itchiness, hunger or sensitivity — which are all messages about how we need to change the way we live to keep the body in its natural harmony and grace.

How we use our senses reflects how we view our physical selves. Sexuality is a metaphor for life in many ways and how one uses ones sexual energy is a good indicator of how we view our lives. We must appreciate the simple art of being more sensitive, more aware in the use of our senses and our lives will unfold spiritually in the temple of the body, which links us to the entire world of Nature.

Triangular Forces

'Rangoantaratma'
- Siva Sutra 3.10
(The inner self is the stage.)

Brahma, Vishnu and Shiva together form a triad of forces represented by an equilateral triangle. This triad of forces manifests on every level of our existence, from the physical to the psychological and the spiritual. Brahma, the creative force generates; Vishnu preserves and protects what has been created; and Shiva as the transcendental force dissolves all phenomenal limitations. Their female consorts or Shaktis similarly form a triad of forces represented by an inverted triangle with Kali at the tip and Lakshmi and Saraswati at the two base points.

The triangle exudes its magical forces, forming the basis of various mystical diagrams or *yantras*. The *yantra* can be used as an all-powerful talisman or as an object of concentration and meditation. The triangle represents the triple principle of creation in both its higher and lower manifestations.

A triangle with its apex upwards indicates a broad-based single pointed aspiration, rising from the depths to the height. *Tantra* refers to it as *vahini kona*, the cone of fire, meaning the fire of aspiration, which is burning forever in every *sadhaka's* heart. The triangle with its apex facing downwards is the responding force of Shakti, the Divine grace of the mother, the *yoni* and the origin of all creation.

The most powerful practice is to transform one's body into a *yantra*, in which all *sadhana* can be internalised. The best *yantra* is said to be the human body, which is why the body must be revered in every respect. The abuse of the body, which is a sacred vehicle, merely for the pleasures of the physical world is a kind of blasphemy. We ourselves create most of the illnesses that happen in our bodies. The body is a mirror image of our beliefs, every cell responding to our every thought. The body is our crystallised thought, densified by the power of time and *karma*.

The human body is a beautiful representation of triangular configurations in both man and woman. The woman's *yoni* forms a downward-pointing triangle, creating duality from which she bears a child. A man's *lingam* and testicles form an upward-pointing triangle, making him strive forward, beyond duality. Only when the two triangles join in unison is creation possible, forming the six-pointed star.

The triangle represents every force in our energy fields. Four triangles form a pyramid when fitted together. They have great significance in Egyptian, Incan and Mayan cultures. These are all configurations of the *yantra*. The flame of the fire forms an upward triangle, perhaps the dominant symbol of worship worldwide. Working with triangular forces through the *yantra*, *Tantra* teaches us how to harness all our inner energies and all the forces of Nature.

Shiva's Child-woman

'And let today embrace the past with remembrance and the
future with longing.'
— Kahlil Gibran

Somehow I always managed to have my way, even when facing the restrictive norms of religious *pundits* or priests. One time I was learning the beautiful art of honouring *agni*, the fire, through the simple *homa* or fire offering. During my stay at Kanatal, I sought permission to celebrate my first fire offering to Lord Shiva on His hilltop temple at some 8,500 feet. I was really pushing my luck as I wanted to perform the *homa* in isolation at the midnight hour.

The villagers and the temple priest knew me well enough to allow me the privilege. The day began with great excitement — collecting all the necessary articles for the *puja*, reading through my script, which I had prepared along with the translations of the Sanskrit *shlokas* and *mantras* I had chosen to use for the occasion. At about half past nine, I stepped out and looked up into the brilliant night sky, raising my hands to Lord Shiva for His blessings. Lo and behold, through the floodlit sky came a powerful star, shooting its way towards the field right in front of me, leaving behind it a trail blaze of bright pink. I was rooted to the ground, awestruck by its sheer brilliance.

We trooped up the hill, a vertical climb, sustained by the clear, crisp air of the October sky. The priest helped me set up the *havan kund* for the fire ceremony and discreetly left me to brave the night. Sitting inside the temple, I prayed in silence and paid obeisance to Lord Shiva, seeking His blessings.

Just short of the midnight hour, my surroundings became steeped in an eerie silence with a visible blinking of lights on the far away mountains across from me. I struck up a match and lit up the wood. Making my offerings with the necessary oblations, the fire seemed to connect with the fiery passions of Nature's energies, its flames rising to magnificent heights, singing fiery praises to my Rudra Lord, Shiva Shankara.

During my *mantra japa*, time seemed to carry me to another space, losing myself to the ethereal world surrounding me. It was simply magical! Then, with the shying away of the embers, ordinary reality seemed to creep back on me, dragging me out of my reverie to the voices of my chauffeur scrambling uphill in the early hour of the new morning. Bless him, for he was always so patient with my madness for Shiva.

To me spirituality is about transcending all concepts and beliefs and directly experiencing for oneself the ineffable truth! Not ever advocating any gullibility, but encouraging a deep questioning, I continued in my quest until as a *seeker*, I had genuinely found my own personal answers to most of my questions, creating an awareness that could never be taken away from me.

My teachers acknowledged that the *"truth* is yours already! Be your own teacher to begin with; you already have the lamp within you. Light it and walk on without fear!" I imbibed this message and learned to challenge my fears, which would often melt away once I did so.

Discovering the beautiful 'art' of spiritual practice means to do what you feel needs to be done, without becoming too holy about it. Fasting, vigils, the study of the scriptures, renouncing possessions and worldly pleasures, are only the means but not the end. Perfection is not to be found in them directly, but may be gradually experienced through them as an approach. The secret is to remember that you are already perfect and that spirituality is a process of discovering this remarkable fact and moving on. Our perfection is in this flow.

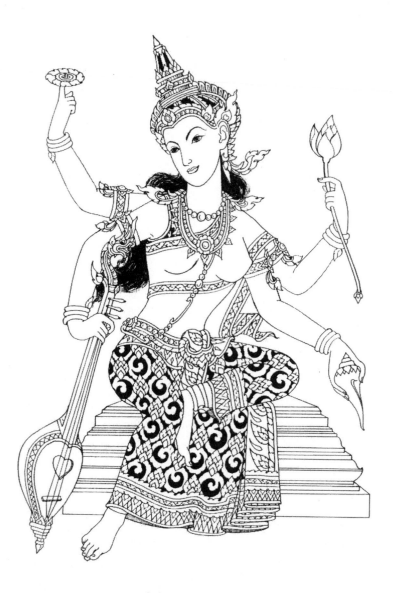

Kamakhya and Beyond

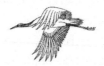

I Am Guided to Kamakhya

'If one having searched it out realises one self here, one gains all
true desires and freedom to move as one desires (*kamachara*) in
all the worlds.'
— *Chandogya Upanishad VIII.1.6*

I was flying to Kamakhya Devi, the most famous of the goddess-
temples, in Guwahati, in the north-eastern state of Assam in India.
I was travelling with the *anugraha*, the blessings of my Mevlana — 'May
Kamakhya-Kamakshi, the Supreme Goddess dispense her power of
vision upon you.' It was also an important personal journey because
Guwahati was my place of birth that I had not returned to since my
family moved away when I was a small child.

Descending down in altitude, the verdant hills came into my view
from the window by my seat. Peering down, my naked eyes searched
for her from the skies, scanning the vastness of the Earth below. The
Kamakhya temple was not to be seen, I could only feel her draw me
into her powerful fold, and the very vibrations were racing through
my being.

An anxiety, nervousness and excitement gripped me. Adding to
this emotional upheaval were man-made fears of a mechanical failure
on the plane. Yes, the announcement system on the flight seemed to
have failed, as the air-hostess's voice was abruptly cut off. Strange
shudders in the cabin brought about a queasy hush to the edgy silence
of the passengers.

Suddenly, all fear released its grip over me. I was open to accept the wishes of Yamadeva, the Lord of Death, if that was the case. The concern for the pain experienced by my near and dear ones all took on an expression of duality. But there were no such plans. The technical problems fixed themselves and the voice of the hostess flowed once more, announcing our approach to Mother Earth.

My tryst with Kamakhya was beginning to unfold for me. Surely for me it was even more emotional because after four decades I was finally returning back to my place of birth. I was coming to terms with the *samskaras* of Kamakhya that remained deep within me. Though I was born in Kamakhya, as my grandparents were living on a tea plantation in Assam, I was not of local descent and we soon moved away from the region, never to return. This left a mystery about my place of birth and I was coming back to understand it — life's experiences having drawn me into their cesspools of happiness, sorrow, love and anguish.

A balmy breeze welcomed me at the airport and I was relieved to see a held up placard read, 'Shambhavi'. I was driven to the guesthouse where I was staying, having been offered the graciousness of the presiding Chief Minister, Shri Tarun Gogoi, through a personal letter of introduction from my *sadhaka*-friend, Prof. Lokesh Chandraji. The drive allowed me to take in the terrain, the tall palms and bamboos calming my senses. The guesthouse was nestled on the banks of the Brahmaputra, the largest and the most masculine of India's rivers, its vast expanse flowing by steadily and relentlessly. Ushered to my room on the higher floor, I was exuberant at the sight before me.

The hues of pink tones of the acacia tree interlaced with the orange flame of the *gulmohur* wafting in the breeze, filtered my gaze on this beautiful, lush little island with an ancient citadel seeking recognition through the dark foliage. The island believed to be the world's smallest human-inhabited river island, holds in its heart a special temple of Shiva and Uma Parvati.

Shiva-Shakti's watchful gaze was trained on me, granting a celestial blessing! The flush of sheer joy sprang from within me. Showering, I sheathed myself in cream and gold, the traditional *dhoti* ensemble from south India, stepping out with excitement and a hint of anxiety for my *darshan* at the temple. I was ready for my visit to the goddesses at the Kamakhya temple.

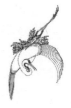

The Swirling Energies at Kamakhya Temple

'Om klim Kamakhya Devyai namah!'

Having arrived at the lotus feet of Kamakhya, at her *yonisthana*, my whole being seemed to transform itself, experiencing the calm composure of a *sadhaka*, all traces of nervousness and anxiety washed away with the earthly residues in the purifying ritual with water, the *kund*, the holy pond.

My feet finding safety on the dark steps led me into the darkness of her earthly *garbha*, her womb-like cave, dim except for the dull strain of the *diya*, preferring not to entirely permeate the darkness within, removing me from the confines of the worldly darkness around.

There was a sound of the gently flowing waters, keeping the moisture within, the very essence of all life. Yet flowing through me was a stream of compassion and gentle strength, a crystal clarity within the deeper recesses of my subtle consciousness, lowering the self in a humility to my knees, placing my hands through the flow of life, caressing in deep reverence the goddess's form bejewelled in flowers and red and gold, the essence of *ittar* and incense impregnating the stillness in the air and in my mind and heart with her supreme activity

Sphura! Sphura, shooting forth the pure unbroken, continuous lightning force, which comes from her *shakti*, She even renders Shiva totally still, having reduced Lord Brahma and Vishnu to servitude. Clearly no one can challenge her!

She brought my heartbeat to a stop, the stoic silence creating a new birth for me beyond this human realm of strife and sorrow.

I sat in the stillness of her deeper silence, lost to her manifold blessings for some 20 minutes, which seemed to open out on to eternity. She seemed to have arrested the oncoming flow of pilgrims to have me for herself! I had requests to make for my Mevlana — the answers arising from my heart to work towards manifesting her truths, to create a happier, peaceful world.

I will never know whether this was the Mother Goddess or my inner voice or simply a manifestation of my deeper thoughts. Time will unravel the truth of this voice, for now I was content in my own realities and bowed in revered silence to her manifold magnitude, withdrawing myself from the sanctity of her all-pervasive benevolence.

Paying obeisance to the head priest, I wandered through a narrow lane, being drawn by an unknown calling. Soon a clearing appeared with a small pond, its whirlpools drawing me into their swirling depths. A strange feeling filled my inner being, when through the concentric circles of energy appeared a huge turtle, its eyes a transparency of grey-green wisdom. The turtle stared into the depths of my soul, probing my very presence at the feet of Kamakhya.

An eeriness came over me, for prior to my journey to Kamakhya I had begun to have turtles appearing in my meditations. In one vision I saw a green turtle at my Mevlana's home, which I had never visited, along with a stone layout and a huge easy chair placed in a large room overlooking a vast expanse of Nature. On mentioning this apparition to my Mevlana, he confirmed its authenticity as his meditation hall. Next I began to see huge turtles; their distinct eyes would haunt me for a long time.

My inner quest to reach out with my experiences to my master drew me into long conversations, surpassing all time and space over the phone, sharing the ecstasy of my experiences, maybe seeking his reassurance and blessings as well.

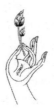

Butterflies Symbolise My Transformation

The Greek word for both 'soul' and 'butterfly' is psyche, and it was once believed that human souls assumed the form of butterflies while they searched for a new incarnation. Butterflies through all the ancient civilisations have maintained their importance as a symbol of the soul and its rebirth, literally representing the 'door of the east', in the Dakota traditions, from which direction appears the splendour of dawn, the dwelling place of the great mystery.

The second day at Guwahati drew me once again into the deeper confines of Devi Kamakhya along with the Mahavidya Goddess's *lila*, their Divine play still ensuing. I first took a boat into the midst of the Brahmaputra to offer myself again to Shiva and Uma Parvati at their island abode.

Nature and its gentle creatures seem to guide me to Shiva's feet, for as I alighted on the island, a black kid goat came upto me, nudging me gently. I stopped to feed it a plantain, which it ceremoniously nibbled at and continued to nudge my sides deeper, leading the way up the flight of stairs. I followed in silence, my heart beginning to flutter. I entered the confines of Shiva's powerful *lingam*, resting deep in a cave. While my being was taking in the intoxication of his masculine energies, there was a heavy presence all of his own!

I seemed to notice on the walls strange depictions of the scorpion, I couldn't seem to draw from this relevance, till sitting in silence and taking in the powers that rested, I suddenly sensed something crawl up to my sides. Looking down, I saw this black scorpion moving alongside my leg. Most certainly a fear crept into my being. What was this cosmic play trying to unfold for me? No sooner had the fear moved away, I settled down to my fate at Shiva's feet. He was impossible at times!

As I stepped into the bright sunshine of the Monday of a *Soma Amavasya*, the fear of life and death was well rewarded with a multitude of beautiful butterflies encircling me. I tried to capture their magic on film, only to realise they drew a blank in the positive, which left me thinking, were they for real? I circumambulated around the temple and strolled over to the other side of the island, in the depths of a heavenly reverie.

The hooting of the boat brought me out of this reverie, drawing me down the flight of stairs. My eyes warmed to the gentle sight of the kid goat, walking up to acknowledge my pilgrimage. I sat down to its gentle nuzzle in my lap.

The afternoon took me to the hill once again where the Ten Wisdom Goddessess unfolded their forms in deep caves, in manifestations of rock formations. Chhinnamasta Ma drew me into her dark, deep recesses, the flight of steep stone steps being all of two inches wide, well oiled through years of obeisance. Bhairavi led me to her magical self, having me escorted out of her cave by a huge wild chameleon. The creatures I was scared of seemed to cross my path here.

I was ascending a flight of stairs out in the midst of nowhere, when once again I seemed to be encircled by about two dozen large black butterflies, which seemed like baby bats to me. They brushed my bare arms. Looking around I realised there was not a single flower or flowering shrub in sight. They led me to the doors of Ma Dhumavati, my wonderful grandmother goddess.

Making my way to Kamakhya Devi, I spent over an hour-and-a-half in quiet meditation by her side, praying for each of the wish lists I had carried from my near and dear ones. The *yantras* in my book of *Tantric Yoga and the Wisdom Goddesses* found their *shaktis* being charged. I made an offering of a coconut from my Mevlana, placing it at all the *devi's* feet, applying their markings of red *sindoor*.

The power of Ma Tara and Kali were anxiously awaiting me. Only when the time is right will she allow you into her deeper confines. For having traversed the tiny path before, my eyes never caught sight of either *shaktisthanas*, places. The doors to Tara were closed, but a child came upto me and asked me to open the doors and go inside.

Quite taken aback, I did unlock the doors, only to be embraced by her awesome energy. I fell to my knees with folded hands, making an offering of two lotuses. Yes, I carried a pair of lotuses to make an offering to each goddess — one from my Mevlana and one from me. I applied the *tilak* of *sindoor* from her feet to the offering of the coconut and my forehead. She seemed to want me to be alone with her to the timing worked out by her magical clock.

I stepped out of Ma Tara's magical embrace into the enigmatic fold of Maha Kali! The residing priest saw me and bowed away to the outer vicinity, as if on instructions from her. I stood alone rooted to the Earth around her very presence. My whole being was reduced to a tremulous offering at her feet. Quivering, I placed the pair of lotuses, taking in the blessings with the mark of the *sindoor*, writing its passion in the brilliance of red, bringing to my mind the play of *Rakta Kali*, the Red Kali!

Emotions seemed to heighten their play in my human body, it being too much for me to take within the span of a few hours. I still had to make my way up to the top of the hill to Ma Bhuvaneshvari. She had a gentleness emanating from her; actually calming my nerves was a light breeze wafting over me to the flutter of more butterflies. But these seemed of gentler hues and paler tones. I made a wish and reached out my arm, hoping for a butterfly to alight upon my bare skin, fulfilling my wish. Ma is always benevolent! The butterflies did alight gently, brushing my skin with a tingling of their beautiful energies.

The bright hues of *sarson*, the mustard flowers, in all their brilliant yellow brought about the grand finale at Ma Bagalamukhi's feet. To her I made the offering of two beautiful yellow silk scarves trimmed with gold tassels, alongwith the pair of lotuses. I stepped outside to light a *diya*, the oil lamp, when suddenly the powerful yoddling sound of women rendered the air with a distinct eeriness. I stood in stoic silence, not allowing my gaze to move away from the flame of the lamp. I deeply sensed the impending call of Ma for a sacrifice.

The sound of the flutter of death to my left was both felt and heard, experiencing the sacrifice of a bird being offered to Ma. I had no choice in this; it was their calling. Of course, the goddesses had contrived this powerful ode to the offering of myself at their feet, acknowledging and lovingly accepting me into their imminent fold.

'Jai Kamakhya Kamakshya!'

Kamarupa Complies with My Deepest Desires

'In this space within the heart are placed both Heaven and Earth, both fire and air, both Sun and Moon, both the lightning and the stars. Whatever is here and whatever is not here, all that is rests within it.'
— *Chandogya Upanishad VIII.1.3*

That night the beautiful strains of a singer's passionate rendition of love drew me back into the throes of worldly existence. Standing in the darkness of the nearing *Kali Raat,* the night of darkness before the A*mavasya,* new Moon, Shiva pulled the strings of my heart yet again, a gentle reminder of my womanly urges.

The pure surge of complete surrender carried my heartbeats across the silent waves of the Brahmaputra, with its plea to Shiva and Parvati, the immortal, transcendental lovers, and a silent prayer rose to my lips from the depths of my heart for happiness and blessings to fill the life of the faceless beautiful voice.

The quest lingers on my lips for a love-wish written in stone. Assam is Kamarupa, the form of desire, and the *devi* is Kamakshi (Sanskrit of Kamakhya) — she who grants the fulfilment of the deepest desires through her glance alone.

'*Om namo Parvati patey har har Mahadeva!*'

My Mevlana guided me to the land of Kamarupa and the *nila parvatas*, the dark blue hills, frequented by the hosts of *siddhas*, which they say is the 'playground of the goddess, the supreme auspicious secret womb of Goddess Kameshwari being the root of the world!'

The east is where light ushers itself in through the first rays of the sunrise. The northeast, where light makes its first intimation, is the direction of Brahman, from where the Divine influence of the Shiva force permeates our spatial Earth. All meditation is best performed when oriented, facing either the east or the northeast, bearing these influences. The northeast of India has the wonder of Kamakhya as well, which a few pilgrims visit, though the ancient teachings laud it as the supreme seat of the goddess.

It was the most auspicious night of the *Soma Amavasya*, falling on a Monday, that lulled me into a deep sleep, with the contentment of a zillion blessings. In the dawn of the new Moon, I was blessed with the *darshan*, appearance, of Ma Kali at the foot of my bed only to be followed by my Mevlana standing on the left side of my bed. I drew from their blessings into the deeper recesses of my heart, losing myself to the magic of their wonder!

I strongly felt the calling of the Dasha Mahavidya Goddesses, feeling there was still some unfinished work to do with their transformative energies. Shiva and Devi were carrying me forward into another world and another life, another magical and transformative turn in the inner journey!

'Jai Gurudeva! Jai Ma Guru!'